PSORIATIC ARTHRITIS DIET COOKBOOK FOR BEGINNERS

Simple, Anti-Inflammatory Recipes to Soothe Symptoms and Enhance Well-being

Kingsley Klopp

To show our appreciation for your purchase, we're delighted to offer you these special bonuses as a heartfelt thank you.

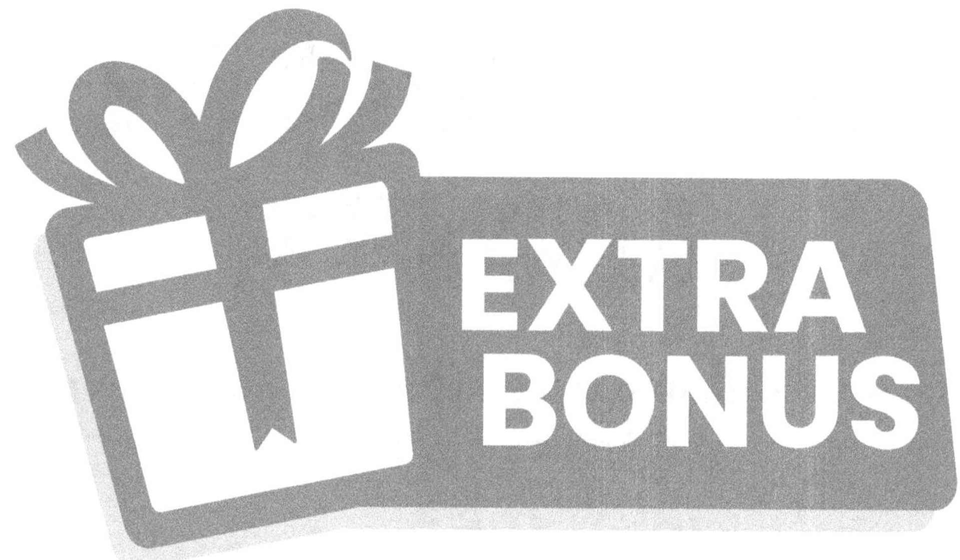

1. A Food Tracker Journal
2. Downloadable E-BOOK featuring full-color images of finished recipes

Table of Contents

Soup & Stew

Snacks & Desserts

Important Note

As you set out on this delicious exploration through our **"Psoriatic Arthritis Diet Cookbook,"** it's important to remember that each dish has been crafted not only with flavor in mind but also with the intent to help soothe and manage the symptoms of psoriatic arthritis through diet. However, it's essential to recognize that each individual's journey with psoriatic arthritis is unique, and what works for one may not work for all. As you try out the recipes in this cookbook, we encourage you to listen to your body and adjust the ingredients according to your personal dietary needs and preferences. Your body is your most reliable guide, and it will let you know what works best for you.

Moreover, we understand that navigating dietary choices can sometimes be as complex as the flavors in your kitchen. If you ever find yourself unsure or in need of guidance on how to tailor these recipes to better suit your health requirements, please consult with your healthcare provider. They can offer personalized advice that complements the nutritional strategies outlined in this book.

Please also note that the nutritional information provided with each recipe is approximate. Variations in specific ingredients used or changes in portion sizes can affect the nutritional value of each dish. We strive to provide accurate estimations to help you make informed decisions about what you eat, but these numbers should be used as a guideline rather than an exact science.

Furthermore, If our cookbook has brought joy to your kitchen and table, we'd be thrilled to hear about your experiences in an Amazon review. On the flip side, if you stumble upon any hiccups while exploring our recipes, don't hesitate to get in touch at kloppkingsley@gmail.com. We're here to support your cooking journey every step of the way.

We've poured love, care, and a dash of creativity into every page of this cookbook, hoping to bring warmth and wellness into your kitchen. May these recipes bring you not only relief and health but also joy and satisfaction at your dining table. Remember, you're not just feeding your body; you're nourishing your spirit and embracing a life of vibrant health.

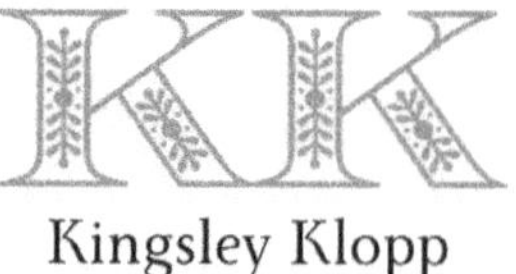

Kingsley Klopp

Introduction

Imagine waking up every morning, not with the usual stiffness or minor aches that come from a restless night or an overenthusiastic workout, but with a pain that gnaws deep into your joints and a skin that itches and flakes, often leaving you more exhausted than when you went to bed. This isn't just a bad day; this is a reality for many dealing with psoriatic arthritis, a chronic autoimmune disease that doesn't just affect the joints but also the skin, and indeed, the entire body. But what if I told you that while psoriatic arthritis might be a part of your life, it doesn't have to dictate the quality of it? Yes, there are the doctor visits, the treatments, and medications. But amidst all these, there's a powerful, yet often overlooked ally waiting to be tapped into – your diet.

Welcome to the **"Psoriatic Arthritis Diet Cookbook for Beginners,"** your first step towards transforming the way you eat in a way that not only complements your medical treatments but might also alleviate some of the symptoms associated with psoriatic arthritis. This book is more than just a collection of recipes; it's a new lens through which to view your condition and your lifestyle. Now, you might wonder, "Can what I eat really make a difference?" The answer is a resounding "Yes." While there is no magic diet cure for psoriatic arthritis, numerous studies and countless testimonies have highlighted the profound impact that certain foods can have on reducing inflammation, one of the key players in autoimmune reactions. Our journey through this cookbook will introduce you to anti-inflammatory foods that are not just healthy, but also delicious, easy to prepare, and perfect for your everyday meals. Think about the last time you enjoyed a meal that made you feel good both inside and out. That's the feeling we aim to replicate with every recipe in this book. From breakfast to dinner, and even those crucial snacks in between, each recipe has been crafted with beginners in mind. Whether you're new to the kitchen or just new to cooking with these particular goals, you'll find dishes here that suit your skill level and your taste buds. But this cookbook offers more than just recipes; it's packed with practical advice on how to shop, cook, and eat in a way that's mindful of your psoriatic arthritis. We'll explore which foods to embrace and which to avoid to help manage your symptoms. You'll learn about the hidden sources of inflammation lurking in common foods and discover nutritious alternatives that can help to balance your immune system rather than provoking it.

So, whether you're picking up this book for yourself or for someone you care about, know that within these pages lies more than hope; there's a plan. A plan to eat well, feel better, and live the vibrant life you deserve, despite having psoriatic arthritis. Let's turn the page together and start this delicious, healthful journey.

Chapter 1: The Basics of Psoriatic Arthritis

What is Psoriatic Arthritis?

Psoriatic arthritis (PsA) is a chronic inflammatory condition that combines the symptoms of arthritis and psoriasis, two diseases that can severely impact a person's quality of life. It's more than just a physical ailment; it's a life-altering journey that many people endure, often filled with pain, frustration, and the quest for understanding and relief.

The Origins and History of Psoriatic Arthritis

Psoriatic arthritis has been recognized for centuries, although it was not always understood in the way we know it today. The connection between skin and joint diseases has intrigued medical scholars since ancient times. The first documented descriptions of psoriasis can be traced back to ancient Greece, where the Greek physician Hippocrates wrote about a skin condition resembling psoriasis. However, it wasn't until the 19th and early 20th centuries that medical professionals began to differentiate between psoriasis and other skin conditions like leprosy.

The specific link between psoriasis and arthritis was not clearly established until the early 20th century. In 1818, British dermatologist Robert Willan described the skin manifestations of psoriasis in detail, but it was the pioneering work of scientists in the 20th century that brought the relationship between psoriasis and arthritis into focus. The term "psoriatic arthritis" was officially coined in the mid-20th century, marking a significant milestone in understanding this complex disease.

Development Over Time

As medical science advanced, so did our understanding of psoriatic arthritis. Early research was primarily focused on observing the clinical presentations and patterns of the disease. It became clear that psoriatic arthritis was not just a subset of rheumatoid arthritis, as once thought, but a distinct disease with its own unique characteristics and mechanisms.

By the late 20th century, advances in immunology and genetics began to shed light on the underlying causes of psoriatic arthritis. Researchers discovered that PsA is an autoimmune disorder, where the body's immune system mistakenly attacks its own tissues, leading to inflammation in the joints and skin. This discovery was crucial, as it opened the door to new treatment approaches that specifically target the immune system.

The Emotional Impact

Living with psoriatic arthritis is a deeply personal experience, often fraught with emotional highs and lows. The physical pain and discomfort are just the tip of the iceberg. The disease can be relentless, affecting one's ability to perform everyday tasks, enjoy hobbies, and maintain relationships. The visible skin lesions of psoriasis can lead to self-consciousness, anxiety, and depression, compounding the emotional burden of the disease. Many people with psoriatic arthritis describe feeling isolated and misunderstood. It's a condition that is not always visible to others, leading to a lack of awareness and empathy from those who haven't experienced it. This invisibility can be one of the most challenging aspects to cope with, as it often requires individuals to constantly explain and justify their pain and limitations.

Modern Understanding and Treatments

Today, the treatment landscape for psoriatic arthritis has dramatically improved, offering hope and relief to those affected. The development of biologic therapies, which specifically target the molecules involved in the inflammatory process, has revolutionized the management of PsA. These medications can significantly reduce symptoms, improve joint function, and enhance the quality of life for many patients. Despite these advancements, there is still no cure for psoriatic arthritis. Treatment focuses on managing symptoms and preventing long-term joint damage. This ongoing journey requires a comprehensive approach that includes medication, physical therapy, lifestyle changes, and emotional support.

Looking Ahead

The story of psoriatic arthritis is still being written. Researchers continue to explore the genetic and environmental factors that contribute to the disease, seeking to unlock new and more effective treatments. Advocacy and awareness efforts are crucial in supporting those with PsA, helping to reduce stigma and improve understanding. For those living with psoriatic arthritis, the journey can be daunting, but it is also one of resilience and strength. Every day, individuals with PsA overcome challenges and continue to live their lives to the fullest. By sharing stories, supporting one another, and staying informed, we can foster a community of hope and empowerment.

Symptoms and Diagnosis of Psoriatic Arthritis

Symptoms of Psoriatic Arthritis

Psoriatic arthritis presents a wide range of symptoms, which can vary significantly from person to person. The symptoms can develop slowly over time or come on suddenly, and they often fluctuate between periods of flare-ups and remission. Here are the primary symptoms to watch for:

1. **Joint Pain and Stiffness**
   - Pain: One of the hallmark symptoms of PsA is pain in the joints. This pain can affect any joint in the body, but it commonly targets the knees, ankles, fingers, and toes. The pain can range from mild to severe and often worsens with activity.
   - Stiffness: Many people with PsA experience joint stiffness, especially in the morning or after periods of inactivity. This stiffness can last for more than 30 minutes and may improve with movement.
2. **Swelling and Tenderness**
   - Swollen Joints: Inflammation caused by PsA can lead to visible swelling in the affected joints. This swelling can cause the joints to appear puffy or enlarged.
   - Tenderness: The affected joints may also be tender to the touch, making everyday activities like gripping objects or walking difficult.
3. **Dactylitis (Sausage Fingers or Toes)**
   - This condition is characterized by severe swelling of the fingers or toes, causing them to resemble sausages. Dactylitis is a distinctive feature of PsA and can be particularly painful and debilitating.
4. **Enthesitis**
   - Enthesitis refers to inflammation at the sites where tendons or ligaments attach to the bone, known as entheses. Common sites for enthesitis include the Achilles tendon, the bottoms of the feet, and the areas around the elbows and knees. This inflammation can cause significant pain and discomfort.
5. **Nail Changes**
   - Many individuals with PsA experience changes in their nails. These changes can include pitting (small dents or depressions in the nail surface), discoloration, thickening, and separation of the nail from the nail bed (onycholysis).
6. **Psoriasis Skin Lesions**
   - People with PsA typically have psoriasis, a skin condition that causes red, scaly patches known as plaques. These plaques can appear anywhere on the body but are commonly found on the scalp, elbows, and knees.

7. Fatigue

- Chronic fatigue is a common symptom of PsA. This fatigue is often profound and can interfere with daily activities, making it difficult to maintain a normal routine.

8. Reduced Range of Motion

- Inflammation and joint damage can lead to a reduced range of motion in the affected joints. Over time, this can contribute to disability and impact the quality of life.

Diagnosis of Psoriatic Arthritis

Diagnosing psoriatic arthritis can be challenging due to its variable presentation and overlap with other conditions, such as rheumatoid arthritis and osteoarthritis. However, early and accurate diagnosis is essential for managing the disease effectively and preventing joint damage. The diagnostic process typically involves a combination of clinical evaluation, medical history, imaging studies, and laboratory tests.

1. **Clinical Evaluation**
   - Physical Examination: A thorough physical examination by a healthcare provider is the first step in diagnosing PsA. The doctor will assess the joints for signs of swelling, tenderness, and reduced range of motion. They will also examine the skin for psoriasis lesions and check the nails for any changes.
   - Symptom Review: The doctor will ask about the patient's symptoms, including the onset, duration, and severity of joint pain, stiffness, and swelling. They will also inquire about fatigue and other systemic symptoms.
2. **Medical History**
   - Family History: A detailed medical history, including any family history of psoriasis or psoriatic arthritis, can provide valuable clues. PsA tends to run in families, suggesting a genetic component to the disease.
   - Personal History: Information about the patient's personal history of psoriasis, previous joint problems, and other medical conditions can help in making a diagnosis.
3. **Imaging Studies**
   - X-rays: X-rays of the affected joints can help identify characteristic changes associated with PsA, such as joint erosion, new bone formation, and changes in the shape of the bones.
   - MRI and Ultrasound: These imaging techniques provide more detailed images of the joints and soft tissues. They can detect early signs of inflammation and joint damage that may not be visible on X-rays.

4. Laboratory Tests

- o Blood Tests: While there is no specific blood test for PsA, certain tests can help rule out other conditions and support the diagnosis. These tests may include:
    - Erythrocyte Sedimentation Rate (ESR) and C-Reactive Protein (CRP): These markers indicate inflammation in the body and are often elevated in individuals with PsA.
    - Rheumatoid Factor (RF) and Anti-Cyclic Citrullinated Peptide (anti-CCP): These tests are used to rule out rheumatoid arthritis, as they are typically negative in PsA patients.
    - HLA-B27: This genetic marker is sometimes present in individuals with PsA, particularly those with axial involvement (spine and pelvis).

5. Differential Diagnosis

- o Because PsA shares symptoms with other types of arthritis, a differential diagnosis is crucial. The healthcare provider will carefully consider other potential diagnoses, such as rheumatoid arthritis, osteoarthritis, gout, and ankylosing spondylitis, to ensure an accurate diagnosis.

Receiving a diagnosis of psoriatic arthritis can be an emotional and transformative experience. For many, it brings a sense of relief and validation after months or even years of unexplained symptoms and uncertainty. Finally having a name for their condition can be empowering and a crucial first step toward effective management. However, a diagnosis can also evoke feelings of fear, anxiety, and sadness. The realization of living with a chronic, lifelong condition is daunting, and the prospect of managing symptoms and preventing joint damage can be overwhelming. It is essential for individuals to have access to emotional support and resources to help them navigate this challenging time.

Common Triggers and Flares of Psoriatic Arthritis

What Are Flares?

Flares in psoriatic arthritis are periods when symptoms become more intense and debilitating. During a flare, individuals may experience increased joint pain, stiffness, swelling, and fatigue. Flares can vary in duration and severity, ranging from mild discomfort to severe, immobilizing pain. Recognizing the triggers that precipitate these flares is crucial for managing PsA effectively.

Common Triggers of Psoriatic Arthritis Flares

1. **Stress**
   - Emotional and Physical Stress: Stress, whether emotional or physical, is a significant trigger for many individuals with PsA. Emotional stress can arise from various life events such as work pressures, family issues, or financial concerns. Physical stress includes trauma or injury to the body, which can exacerbate inflammation and trigger a flare.
   - Impact: Stress affects the immune system, leading to increased inflammation. For someone with PsA, this can mean heightened symptoms and more frequent flares.

2. **Infections**
   - Viral and Bacterial Infections: Infections such as the flu, common cold, strep throat, or even dental infections can trigger PsA flares. The immune system's response to fighting off infections can inadvertently cause increased inflammation in the joints and skin.
   - Impact: During an infection, the body's immune response can trigger or worsen psoriatic arthritis symptoms, leading to more severe joint pain and skin lesions.

3. **Weather Changes**
   - Cold and Damp Weather: Many individuals with PsA report that cold, damp weather can worsen their symptoms. Changes in barometric pressure can also affect joint pain and stiffness.
   - Impact: Cold and damp conditions can lead to increased joint stiffness and discomfort, making it more challenging to manage daily activities.

4. **Diet and Nutrition**
   - Certain Foods: Some foods are known to trigger inflammation in individuals with PsA. Common culprits include processed foods, sugary snacks, red meat, and dairy products. Foods high in saturated fats, trans fats, and refined sugars can exacerbate symptoms.
   - Impact: Poor dietary choices can lead to increased inflammation, causing more frequent and severe flares. Conversely, an anti-inflammatory diet rich in fruits, vegetables, whole grains, and omega-3 fatty acids can help manage symptoms.

5. Alcohol and Smoking

- Alcohol Consumption: Excessive alcohol consumption can trigger PsA flares by increasing inflammation and affecting the immune system. Alcohol can also interact with medications used to treat PsA, reducing their effectiveness.
- Smoking: Smoking is another significant trigger, as it can worsen inflammation and contribute to more severe disease progression.
- Impact: Both alcohol and smoking can lead to increased disease activity, making it essential for individuals with PsA to limit or avoid these substances.

6. Hormonal Changes

- Hormonal Fluctuations: Hormonal changes, particularly in women, can trigger PsA flares. These changes can occur during puberty, pregnancy, menopause, or menstrual cycles.
- Impact: Hormonal fluctuations can affect the immune system and inflammation levels, leading to increased joint pain and other symptoms.

7. Medications

- Certain Medications: Some medications, including those for other conditions, can trigger PsA flares. Nonsteroidal anti-inflammatory drugs (NSAIDs), certain blood pressure medications, and lithium are known to potentially worsen symptoms.
- Impact: It's essential for individuals with PsA to discuss all medications with their healthcare provider to ensure they do not exacerbate their condition.

8. Skin Injuries

- Trauma to the Skin: Known as the Koebner phenomenon, injuries to the skin, such as cuts, scrapes, or sunburn, can trigger psoriasis lesions and, subsequently, PsA flares.
- Impact: Protecting the skin from injuries and treating any wounds promptly can help reduce the risk of flares.

9. Obesity

- Excess Weight: Carrying excess weight puts additional stress on the joints, which can trigger or worsen PsA symptoms.
- Impact: Maintaining a healthy weight through diet and exercise can reduce joint stress and inflammation, helping to manage PsA more effectively.

Managing Triggers and Preventing Flares

Understanding and managing triggers is a crucial aspect of living with psoriatic arthritis. Here are some strategies to help prevent flares:

1. **Stress Management**
   - Techniques: Incorporate stress-reducing techniques into daily life, such as mindfulness meditation, yoga, deep breathing exercises, and regular physical activity.
   - Support: Seek support from friends, family, or mental health professionals to help manage emotional stress.

2. Infection Prevention
- Hygiene: Practice good hygiene, such as regular handwashing, to reduce the risk of infections.
- Vaccinations: Stay up to date with vaccinations, including the flu shot, to help prevent infections.

3. Weather Adaptation
- Dress Appropriately: Wear warm clothing in cold weather to protect joints from the cold.
- Indoor Environment: Use humidifiers to maintain moisture in the air during dry conditions.

4. Dietary Adjustments
- Anti-Inflammatory Diet: Follow a diet rich in anti-inflammatory foods, such as leafy greens, fatty fish, nuts, seeds, and olive oil.
- Avoid Triggers: Identify and avoid specific foods that worsen symptoms.

5. Healthy Lifestyle Choices
- Limit Alcohol: Reduce alcohol consumption or avoid it altogether.
- Quit Smoking: Seek support to quit smoking and reduce exposure to secondhand smoke.

6. Hormonal Management
- Monitor Changes: Keep track of hormonal changes and discuss any symptom changes with a healthcare provider.

7. Medication Management
- Review Medications: Regularly review all medications with a healthcare provider to ensure they do not contribute to flares.
- Follow Prescriptions: Adhere to prescribed treatments and report any side effects promptly.

8. Skin Protection
- Avoid Injuries: Take precautions to avoid skin injuries and treat any wounds promptly.
- Sun Protection: Use sunscreen and protective clothing to prevent sunburn.

9. Weight Management
- Healthy Weight: Maintain a healthy weight through balanced nutrition and regular exercise.

The Emotional Toll of Flares

Experiencing a flare can be emotionally challenging. The sudden onset of intense symptoms can disrupt daily life, causing frustration, anxiety, and a sense of helplessness. It's important for individuals with PsA to seek emotional support during these times. Connecting with support groups, talking to mental health professionals, and sharing experiences with loved ones can provide comfort and encouragement.

Key Nutrients for Joint Health in Psoriatic Arthritis

Omega-3 Fatty Acids
Sources:
- Fatty fish (salmon, mackerel, sardines, tuna)
- Flaxseeds and flaxseed oil
- Chia seeds
- Walnuts
- Algal oil (for those who prefer plant-based sources)

Benefits: Omega-3 fatty acids are renowned for their anti-inflammatory properties. They help reduce the production of inflammatory cytokines and enzymes that can damage joints. Regular consumption of omega-3s has been shown to decrease joint pain and stiffness in individuals with arthritis, including PsA.

Incorporation:
- Aim to eat fatty fish at least twice a week.
- Add ground flaxseeds or chia seeds to smoothies, yogurt, or oatmeal.
- Snack on a handful of walnuts or use walnut oil in salad dressings.

Vitamin D
Sources:
- Sunlight exposure (helps the body produce vitamin D)
- Fatty fish (salmon, mackerel, sardines)
- Fortified foods (milk, orange juice, cereals)
- Egg yolks
- Supplements (if needed, after consulting with a healthcare provider)

Benefits: Vitamin D is essential for bone health and helps regulate the immune system. It promotes calcium absorption, which is crucial for maintaining strong bones and reducing the risk of fractures. Adequate vitamin D levels can help mitigate the progression of PsA and improve overall joint health.

Incorporation:
- Spend time outdoors in sunlight, but be mindful of sun protection to avoid skin damage.
- Include vitamin D-rich foods in your diet regularly.
- Consider a vitamin D supplement if dietary intake and sunlight exposure are insufficient.

Calcium
Sources:
- Dairy products (milk, cheese, yogurt)
- Leafy green vegetables (kale, broccoli, bok choy)
- Fortified plant-based milks (almond, soy, oat)
- Sardines and canned salmon (with bones)
- Tofu
- Almonds

Benefits: Calcium is vital for maintaining strong bones and preventing osteoporosis, which can be a concern for individuals with PsA, especially if they are on long-term corticosteroid therapy. Strong bones support healthy joints and reduce the risk of fractures and bone-related complications.

Incorporation:

- Consume dairy or fortified plant-based alternatives daily.
- Include leafy greens in meals regularly.
- Snack on calcium-rich foods like almonds and tofu.

Antioxidants

Sources:

- Fruits and vegetables (berries, citrus fruits, leafy greens, bell peppers)
- Nuts and seeds
- Green tea
- Dark chocolate
- Herbs and spices (turmeric, ginger, garlic)

Benefits: Antioxidants help combat oxidative stress and inflammation, both of which play a role in PsA. Vitamins C and E, as well as selenium and other antioxidant compounds, protect cells from damage and support the immune system in reducing inflammation.

Incorporation:

- Eat a variety of colorful fruits and vegetables every day.
- Enjoy a cup of green tea daily.
- Use antioxidant-rich herbs and spices in cooking.

Protein

Sources:

- Lean meats (chicken, turkey, lean cuts of beef and pork)
- Fish and seafood
- Eggs
- Legumes (beans, lentils, chickpeas)
- Nuts and seeds
- Dairy products
- Plant-based protein sources (tofu, tempeh, edamame)

Benefits: Protein is essential for repairing and maintaining tissues, including muscles and joints. Adequate protein intake supports muscle strength, which is important for joint stability and reducing the strain on affected joints.

Incorporation:

- Include a source of lean protein in every meal.
- Explore plant-based protein options for variety and additional health benefits.
- Use legumes and nuts as snacks or add them to salads and main dishes.

Fiber
Sources:
- Whole grains (oats, quinoa, brown rice, whole wheat)
- Fruits and vegetables
- Legumes (beans, lentils, chickpeas)
- Nuts and seeds

Benefits: Fiber supports overall health by promoting a healthy digestive system, which can indirectly affect inflammation and immune function. A diet high in fiber helps regulate blood sugar levels, which is beneficial for managing PsA and maintaining a healthy weight.

Incorporation:
- Choose whole grains over refined grains.
- Aim to fill half your plate with fruits and vegetables at each meal.
- Include legumes in soups, stews, and salads.

Vitamin C
Sources:
- Citrus fruits (oranges, lemons, grapefruits)
- Berries (strawberries, blueberries, raspberries)
- Bell peppers
- Broccoli
- Brussels sprouts
- Tomatoes
- Kiwi

Benefits: Vitamin C is crucial for collagen production, which is essential for maintaining the integrity of cartilage and connective tissues in the joints. It also acts as an antioxidant, helping to reduce inflammation and support immune function.

Incorporation:
- Snack on citrus fruits and berries.
- Add bell peppers and tomatoes to salads and meals.
- Include vitamin C-rich vegetables like broccoli and Brussels sprouts in your diet.

Vitamin E
Sources:
- Nuts and seeds (almonds, sunflower seeds, hazelnuts)
- Vegetable oils (sunflower, safflower, olive oil)
- Spinach and other leafy greens
- Avocados

Benefits: Vitamin E is a powerful antioxidant that helps protect cells from damage caused by free radicals. It plays a role in reducing inflammation and supporting immune function, which is beneficial for individuals with PsA.

Incorporation:
- Use vegetable oils in cooking and dressings.
- Snack on a handful of nuts and seeds.
- Include spinach and other leafy greens in meals.

Curcumin (Turmeric)
Sources:
- Turmeric spice
- Turmeric supplements (consult a healthcare provider before starting any supplement)

Benefits: Curcumin, the active ingredient in turmeric, has potent anti-inflammatory and antioxidant properties. Studies have shown that curcumin can help reduce joint pain and inflammation in individuals with arthritis.

Incorporation:
- Add turmeric to soups, stews, and curries.
- Make a turmeric latte with warm milk (dairy or plant-based) and a dash of black pepper to enhance absorption.

Selenium
Sources:
- Brazil nuts (an excellent source of selenium)
- Seafood (tuna, sardines, shrimp)
- Eggs
- Sunflower seeds
- Whole grains

Benefits: Selenium is a trace mineral that acts as an antioxidant, helping to reduce inflammation and support immune function. Adequate selenium intake is associated with lower levels of inflammatory markers in the body.

Incorporation:
- Eat a few Brazil nuts daily (be mindful of portion sizes to avoid excessive intake).
- Include seafood in your diet regularly.
- Use sunflower seeds as a topping for salads and yogurt.

Incorporating Key Nutrients into Your Diet
To ensure you are getting all the key nutrients necessary for joint health, focus on a balanced and varied diet. Here are some practical tips:
- Meal Planning: Plan your meals ahead of time to include a variety of nutrient-dense foods. This helps ensure you get a wide range of vitamins and minerals.
- Balanced Meals: Aim to include a source of protein, healthy fats, fiber, and a variety of fruits and vegetables in each meal.
- Healthy Snacking: Choose nutrient-rich snacks like nuts, seeds, fruits, and vegetables to keep your energy levels stable and provide essential nutrients throughout the day.
- Cooking Methods: Opt for cooking methods that preserve the nutrient content of foods, such as steaming, grilling, and baking, rather than frying.
- Supplements: If you find it challenging to get certain nutrients from your diet alone, consider discussing supplements with your healthcare provider.

Anti-Inflammatory Foods for Psoriatic Arthritis

The Role of Diet in Inflammation

Diet plays a crucial role in managing inflammation. Anti-inflammatory foods contain nutrients that can help reduce the production of inflammatory chemicals in the body, support the immune system, and promote overall health. By focusing on these foods, individuals with PsA can potentially alleviate their symptoms and improve their quality of life.

Top Anti-Inflammatory Foods

1. Fatty Fish

Examples: Salmon, mackerel, sardines, tuna, trout

Benefits: Fatty fish are rich in omega-3 fatty acids, particularly EPA and DHA, which have potent anti-inflammatory effects. These fatty acids help reduce the production of inflammatory cytokines and prostaglandins, which are chemicals involved in the inflammatory response.

Incorporation:

- Aim to include fatty fish in your diet at least two to three times per week.
- Try grilling, baking, or broiling fish for a healthy meal.
- Add canned salmon or sardines to salads and sandwiches.

2. Leafy Green Vegetables

Examples: Spinach, kale, Swiss chard, collard greens

Benefits: Leafy greens are packed with vitamins, minerals, and antioxidants that combat inflammation. They are particularly high in vitamin K, which has been shown to help reduce inflammatory markers in the body.

Incorporation:

- Include leafy greens in salads, smoothies, and stir-fries.
- Use spinach or kale as a base for salads or as an addition to soups and stews.
- Sauté Swiss chard or collard greens with garlic and olive oil for a nutritious side dish.

3. Berries

Examples: Blueberries, strawberries, raspberries, blackberries

Benefits: Berries are rich in antioxidants, such as anthocyanins and quercetin, which help reduce inflammation and oxidative stress. They also contain fiber, vitamins, and minerals that support overall health.

Incorporation:

- Add fresh or frozen berries to smoothies, yogurt, or oatmeal.
- Snack on berries throughout the day.
- Use berries as a topping for salads or desserts.

4. Nuts and Seeds

Examples: Almonds, walnuts, flaxseeds, chia seeds, sunflower seeds

Benefits: Nuts and seeds are excellent sources of healthy fats, protein, and fiber. They contain omega-3 fatty acids, particularly in walnuts, flaxseeds, and chia seeds, which have anti-inflammatory properties. They also provide vitamin E, magnesium, and antioxidants that help reduce inflammation.

Incorporation:

- Snack on a handful of nuts or seeds.
- Add flaxseeds or chia seeds to smoothies, yogurt, or oatmeal.
- Use nuts and seeds as a topping for salads and stir-fries.

5. Olive Oil

Benefits: Olive oil, especially extra virgin olive oil, is rich in monounsaturated fats and antioxidants, including oleocanthal, which has anti-inflammatory effects similar to ibuprofen. It helps reduce inflammation and supports heart health.

Incorporation:

- Use olive oil as a primary cooking oil.
- Drizzle olive oil over salads, vegetables, and grains.
- Use olive oil in marinades and dressings.

6. Turmeric

Benefits: Turmeric contains curcumin, a powerful anti-inflammatory and antioxidant compound. Curcumin has been shown to inhibit the activity of inflammatory molecules in the body and reduce symptoms of arthritis.

Incorporation:

- Add turmeric to curries, soups, and stews.
- Make a turmeric latte with warm milk (dairy or plant-based) and a dash of black pepper to enhance absorption.
- Use turmeric in spice blends for seasoning meats and vegetables.

7. Garlic

Benefits: Garlic is known for its anti-inflammatory and immune-boosting properties. It contains sulfur compounds, such as allicin, which help reduce inflammation and support overall health.

Incorporation:

- Add fresh garlic to sauces, soups, and stir-fries.
- Use garlic powder or minced garlic as a seasoning for meats and vegetables.
- Roast whole garlic cloves for a milder, sweeter flavor.

8. Ginger

Benefits: Ginger contains bioactive compounds like gingerol, which have anti-inflammatory and antioxidant effects. It helps reduce inflammation and can alleviate symptoms of arthritis.

Incorporation:
- Add fresh ginger to smoothies, teas, and stir-fries.
- Use ground ginger in baking and cooking.
- Make ginger tea by steeping fresh ginger slices in hot water.

9. Tomatoes

Benefits: Tomatoes are rich in lycopene, an antioxidant that helps reduce inflammation. Cooking tomatoes increases the availability of lycopene, making tomato-based sauces and soups particularly beneficial.

Incorporation:
- Add fresh tomatoes to salads and sandwiches.
- Use canned or fresh tomatoes in soups, stews, and sauces.
- Enjoy tomato juice or gazpacho.

10. Green Tea

Benefits: Green tea is packed with polyphenols, particularly epigallocatechin gallate (EGCG), which have strong anti-inflammatory and antioxidant properties. Regular consumption of green tea can help reduce inflammation and support overall health.

Incorporation:
- Drink green tea daily, either hot or iced.
- Add matcha powder to smoothies, yogurt, or baked goods.
- Use green tea as a base for marinades and broths.

Foods to Avoid for Psoriatic Arthritis

Foods to Avoid

1. Processed and Refined Sugars

Examples: Sodas, candies, pastries, cookies, and other sugary snacks

Impact: Processed and refined sugars can trigger the release of inflammatory cytokines, molecules that promote inflammation in the body. High sugar intake is associated with increased levels of pro-inflammatory markers, which can worsen PsA symptoms.

Avoidance Tips:

- Opt for natural sweeteners like honey or maple syrup in moderation.
- Choose fresh fruits to satisfy sweet cravings.
- Read labels to identify and avoid added sugars in packaged foods.

2. Refined Carbohydrates

Examples: White bread, white rice, pasta, and other refined grains

Impact: Refined carbohydrates have a high glycemic index, leading to rapid spikes in blood sugar levels. These spikes can increase inflammation and contribute to weight gain, which adds stress to the joints.

Avoidance Tips:

- Replace refined grains with whole grains like brown rice, quinoa, and whole wheat bread.
- Choose whole grain pasta or alternative grains like farro and barley.
- Incorporate a variety of fiber-rich vegetables and legumes in meals.

3. Red and Processed Meats

Examples: Beef, pork, lamb, bacon, sausage, hot dogs, and deli meats

Impact: Red and processed meats contain high levels of saturated fats and advanced glycation end products (AGEs), which can increase inflammation. These meats are also linked to higher levels of inflammatory markers in the body.

Avoidance Tips:

- Choose lean protein sources like poultry, fish, and plant-based proteins.
- Limit consumption of red meat and opt for grass-fed or organic options when you do eat it.
- Avoid processed meats and opt for fresh, unprocessed alternatives.

4. Dairy Products

Examples: Milk, cheese, butter, yogurt, and ice cream

Impact: Dairy products can be inflammatory for some people, especially those with a sensitivity to lactose or casein, the protein found in milk. Dairy consumption can lead to increased inflammation and joint pain in individuals with PsA.

Avoidance Tips:

- Try dairy alternatives like almond milk, soy milk, or oat milk.
- Choose dairy-free yogurt and cheese options.
- Experiment with dairy-free recipes to find alternatives that work for you.

5. Fried and Fast Foods

Examples: French fries, fried chicken, doughnuts, and fast food items

Impact: Fried and fast foods are typically high in trans fats, unhealthy saturated fats, and calories, all of which can promote inflammation. These foods can contribute to weight gain and worsen PsA symptoms.

Avoidance Tips:

- Prepare meals at home using healthier cooking methods like baking, grilling, or steaming.
- Choose whole, unprocessed foods over fast food options.
- Use healthy fats like olive oil or avocado oil for cooking.

6. Alcohol

Examples: Beer, wine, spirits, and cocktails

Impact: Excessive alcohol consumption can increase inflammation and interfere with the effectiveness of medications used to treat PsA. Alcohol can also lead to dehydration, which can worsen joint pain and stiffness.

Avoidance Tips:

- Limit alcohol intake and choose non-alcoholic beverages.
- Stay hydrated by drinking plenty of water throughout the day.
- If you do drink alcohol, do so in moderation and choose low-sugar options.

7. Certain Vegetable Oils

Examples: Corn oil, soybean oil, sunflower oil, and other oils high in omega-6 fatty acids

Impact: These vegetable oils contain high levels of omega-6 fatty acids, which can promote inflammation when consumed in excess. A diet high in omega-6 fatty acids and low in omega-3s can lead to an imbalance that exacerbates inflammation.

Avoidance Tips:

- Use oils high in omega-3 fatty acids, such as olive oil, flaxseed oil, and walnut oil.
- Reduce the use of processed foods that contain these oils.
- Balance omega-6 intake with omega-3-rich foods like fatty fish and flaxseeds.

8. Gluten-Containing Foods

Examples: Wheat, barley, rye, and foods made from these grains

Impact: For some individuals, gluten can trigger inflammation and worsen PsA symptoms. This is especially true for those with a sensitivity to gluten or celiac disease.

Avoidance Tips:

- Opt for gluten-free grains like quinoa, rice, and gluten-free oats.
- Read labels to ensure packaged foods are gluten-free.
- Experiment with gluten-free baking and cooking to find suitable alternatives.

9. Nightshade Vegetables

Examples: Tomatoes, eggplants, bell peppers, and potatoes

Impact: Nightshade vegetables contain solanine, a compound that can trigger inflammation in some individuals. While not everyone with PsA will be affected, those who are sensitive to nightshades may experience increased joint pain and stiffness.

Avoidance Tips:

- Monitor your symptoms and see if they improve when you eliminate nightshade vegetables.
- Replace nightshades with other vegetables like leafy greens, broccoli, and carrots.
- Gradually reintroduce nightshades to see if they trigger symptoms.

Further Clarification

Tomatoes and Psoriatic Arthritis

Tomatoes are often included in lists of anti-inflammatory foods because they are rich in antioxidants like lycopene, which has been shown to have anti-inflammatory properties. However, tomatoes belong to the nightshade family, which includes other vegetables like eggplants, bell peppers, and potatoes. Some individuals with psoriatic arthritis report that nightshade vegetables can exacerbate their symptoms.

The Dual Perspective on Tomatoes

Anti-Inflammatory Benefits

Benefits:

- Lycopene: Tomatoes are an excellent source of lycopene, an antioxidant that helps reduce inflammation in the body. Lycopene is more bioavailable when tomatoes are cooked, making tomato-based sauces and soups beneficial.
- Vitamins and Minerals: Tomatoes are also rich in vitamins A and C, which are important for immune function and overall health.

Incorporation:

- Including tomatoes in your diet can provide these anti-inflammatory benefits. You might enjoy them fresh in salads, cooked in sauces, or blended into soups.

Potential Drawbacks for Some Individuals

Concerns:

- Nightshade Sensitivity: Some individuals with psoriatic arthritis may have a sensitivity to nightshade vegetables, which can potentially trigger inflammation and exacerbate symptoms. This is not the case for everyone, but it can be significant for those who are sensitive.

Avoidance:

- If you notice that consuming tomatoes or other nightshade vegetables like eggplants, bell peppers, and potatoes worsens your symptoms, it may be beneficial to limit or avoid them.
- Keeping a food diary can help identify if nightshades are a trigger for your symptoms.

Personalized Approach

Individual Variation

Psoriatic arthritis affects individuals differently, and dietary responses can vary. What works for one person might not work for another. Therefore, it is essential to approach dietary recommendations with flexibility and personalization.

Trial and Observation

- Trial Elimination: Consider eliminating tomatoes and other nightshade vegetables from your diet for a few weeks to see if your symptoms improve.
- Reintroduction: Gradually reintroduce these foods one at a time to observe any changes in your symptoms.

Breakfast Recipes

1. Baked Apple with Cinnamon
Ingredients:
- 4 large apples (such as Honeycrisp or Granny Smith)
- 2 tablespoons honey or maple syrup
- 1 teaspoon ground cinnamon
- 1/4 teaspoon ground nutmeg
- 1/4 cup chopped walnuts (optional)
- 1/4 cup raisins or dried cranberries (optional)

Instructions:
1. Preheat your oven to 350°F (175°C).
2. Core the apples and place them in a baking dish.
3. In a small bowl, mix honey or maple syrup, ground cinnamon, and ground nutmeg.
4. Pour the mixture evenly over the apples.
5. If using, sprinkle chopped walnuts and raisins or dried cranberries over the apples.
6. Cover the baking dish with foil and bake for 25-30 minutes, until the apples are tender.
7. Remove the foil and bake for an additional 5 minutes to allow the top to brown slightly.
8. Serve warm.

Number of Serves: 4
Nutritional Info per Serving:
- Calories: 120
- Protein: 1g
- Carbohydrates: 30g
- Fiber: 5g
- Sugars: 22g
- Fat: 2g (if walnuts are included)

Cooking Time: 35-40 minutes

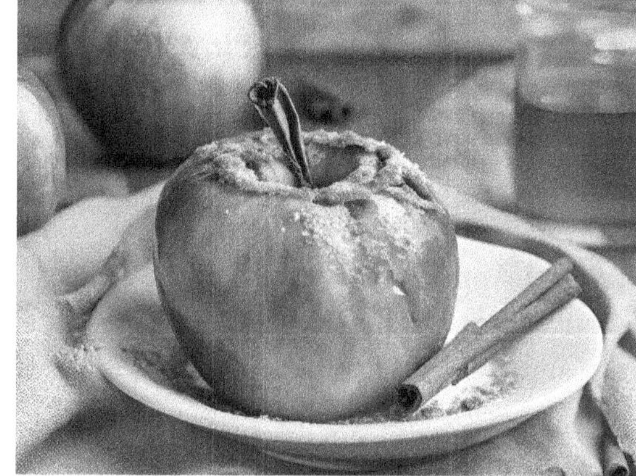

2. Cucumber and Lime Chilled Soup

Ingredients:

- 2 large cucumbers, peeled and chopped
- 1 cup plain Greek yogurt
- 1 clove garlic, minced
- 1/4 cup fresh lime juice
- 1 tablespoon olive oil
- 1/4 cup fresh dill or mint, chopped
- Salt and pepper to taste
- 1/2 cup water (or more for desired consistency)

Instructions:

1. In a blender, combine chopped cucumbers, Greek yogurt, minced garlic, fresh lime juice, olive oil, and fresh dill or mint.
2. Blend until smooth. If the soup is too thick, add water a little at a time until desired consistency is reached.
3. Season with salt and pepper to taste.
4. Chill in the refrigerator for at least 1 hour before serving.
5. Serve cold, garnished with additional dill or mint if desired.

Number of Serves: 4

Nutritional Info per Serving:

- Calories: 90
- Protein: 5g
- Carbohydrates: 10g
- Fiber: 1g
- Sugars: 6g
- Fat: 4g

Cooking Time: 15 minutes (plus chilling time)

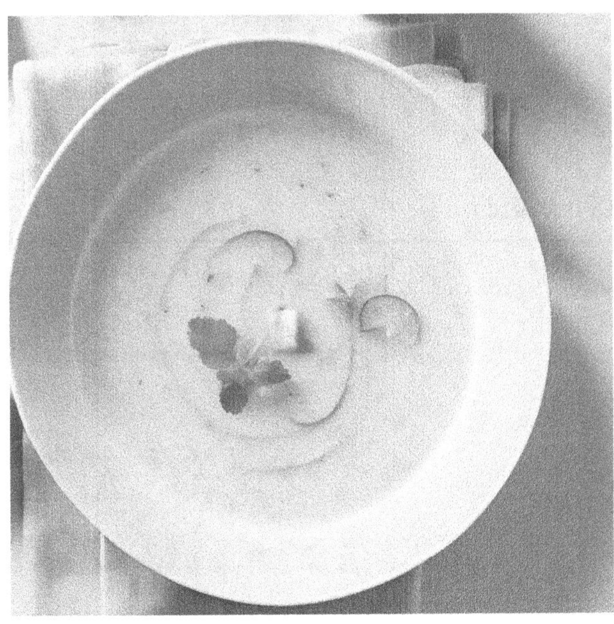

3. Walnut and Pear Baked Oatmeal

Ingredients:

- 2 cups rolled oats
- 1 teaspoon baking powder
- 1 teaspoon ground cinnamon
- 1/2 teaspoon ground nutmeg
- 1/4 teaspoon salt
- 2 cups almond milk (or any milk of choice)
- 1/4 cup maple syrup or honey
- 1 large egg
- 1 teaspoon vanilla extract
- 2 ripe pears, peeled and chopped
- 1/2 cup chopped walnuts

Instructions:

1. Preheat your oven to 375°F (190°C) and grease a 9x9-inch baking dish.
2. In a large bowl, mix together rolled oats, baking powder, ground cinnamon, ground nutmeg, and salt.
3. In another bowl, whisk together almond milk, maple syrup or honey, egg, and vanilla extract.
4. Pour the wet ingredients into the dry ingredients and mix until combined.
5. Fold in the chopped pears and walnuts.
6. Pour the mixture into the prepared baking dish and spread evenly.
7. Bake for 35-40 minutes, until the top is golden brown and the oatmeal is set.
8. Let it cool for a few minutes before serving.

Number of Serves: 6

Nutritional Info per Serving:

- Calories: 220
- Protein: 5g
- Carbohydrates: 34g
- Fiber: 5g
- Sugars: 12g
- Fat: 8g

Cooking Time: 40-45 minutes

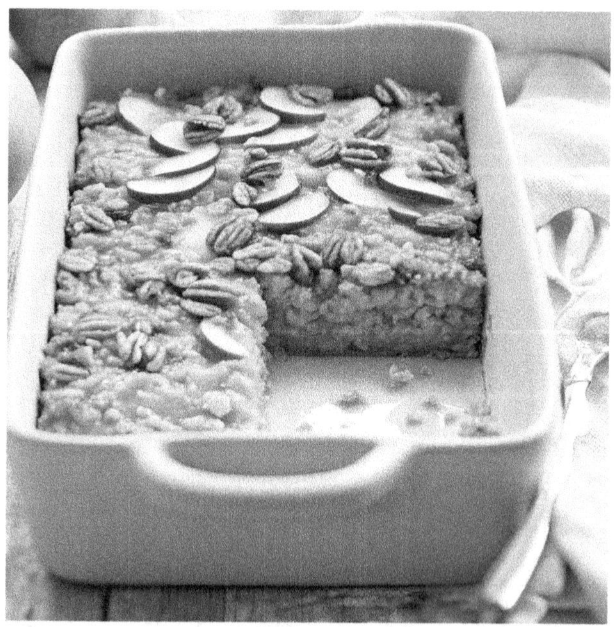

4. Matcha Green Tea

Ingredients:

- 1 teaspoon matcha green tea powder
- 1 cup hot water (not boiling, around 175°F or 80°C)
- Optional: sweetener of choice (honey, agave syrup, etc.)
- Optional: a splash of almond milk or other milk of choice

Instructions:

1. Sift 1 teaspoon of matcha green tea powder into a bowl to remove any lumps.
2. Add a small amount of hot water (about 2 tablespoons) to the bowl and whisk the matcha powder with a bamboo whisk (chasen) or a small regular whisk until it forms a smooth paste.
3. Add the remaining hot water and whisk in a zigzag motion until the tea is frothy.
4. If desired, add sweetener and a splash of milk.
5. Pour into a cup and serve immediately.

Number of Serves: 1

Nutritional Info per Serving:

- Calories: 10 (without sweetener or milk)
- Protein: 0g
- Carbohydrates: 2g
- Fiber: 0g
- Sugars: 0g
- Fat: 0g

Cooking Time: 5 minutes

5. Kale and Avocado Wrap

Ingredients:

- 1 large whole-grain tortilla
- 1 ripe avocado, mashed
- 1 cup kale, finely chopped
- 1 small carrot, grated
- 1/4 cup red bell pepper, thinly sliced
- 2 tablespoons hummus
- 1 tablespoon lemon juice
- 1 teaspoon olive oil

Instructions:

1. In a small bowl, mix the chopped kale with lemon juice and olive oil. Massage the kale for a few minutes until it softens.
2. Lay the tortilla flat and spread the hummus evenly over it.
3. Spread the mashed avocado on top of the hummus.
4. Add the massaged kale, grated carrot, and red bell pepper on top.
5. Roll up the tortilla tightly and slice it in half.
6. Serve immediately.

Number of Serves: 1

Nutritional Info per Serving:

- Calories: 350
- Protein: 8g
- Carbohydrates: 40g
- Fiber: 12g
- Sugars: 4g
- Fat: 20g

Cooking Time: 10 minutes

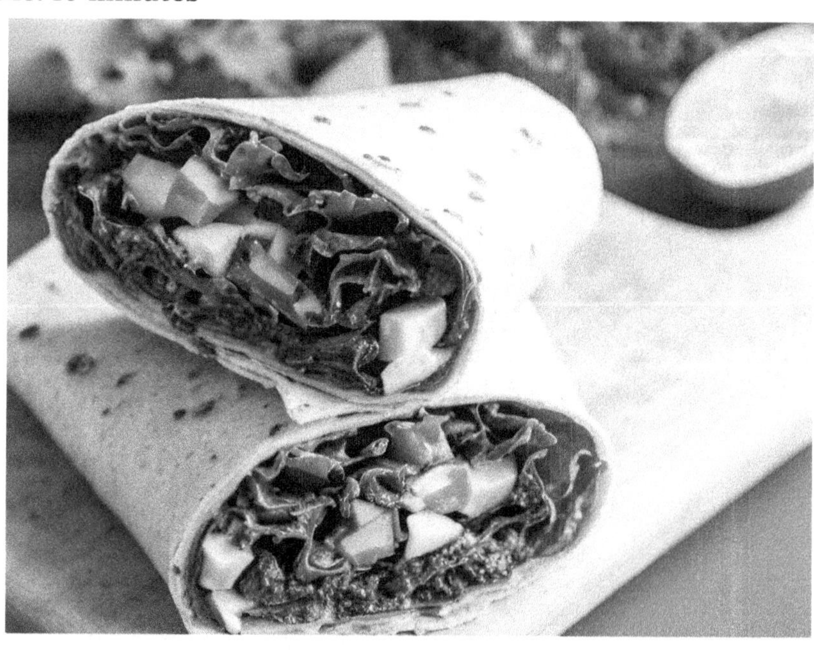

6. Spinach and Mushroom Crepes

Ingredients:

- **For the crepes:**
  - 1/2 cup whole wheat flour
  - 1/2 cup almond milk (or any plant-based milk)
  - 1 large egg
  - 1/4 cup water
  - 1 tablespoon olive oil
- **For the filling:**
  - 1 cup spinach, chopped
  - 1 cup mushrooms, sliced
  - 1 clove garlic, minced
  - 1 tablespoon olive oil

Instructions:

1. **Make the crepes:**
   - In a bowl, whisk together the flour, almond milk, egg, water, and olive oil until smooth.
   - Heat a non-stick skillet over medium heat. Pour about 1/4 cup of batter into the skillet and swirl to coat the bottom. Cook for about 1-2 minutes until the edges start to lift, then flip and cook for another minute. Repeat with remaining batter.
2. **Prepare the filling:**
   - In another skillet, heat olive oil over medium heat. Add garlic and mushrooms, and cook until mushrooms are tender, about 5 minutes. Add spinach and cook until wilted, about 2 more minutes.
3. Assemble the crepes:
   - Place a crepe on a plate, add some of the spinach and mushroom filling, and fold or roll up the crepe. Repeat with the remaining crepes and filling.
   - Serve warm.

Number of Serves: 4

Nutritional Info per Serving:

- Calories: 180
- Protein: 6g
- Carbohydrates: 20g
- Fiber: 3g
- Sugars: 2g
- Fat: 8g

Cooking Time: 30 minutes

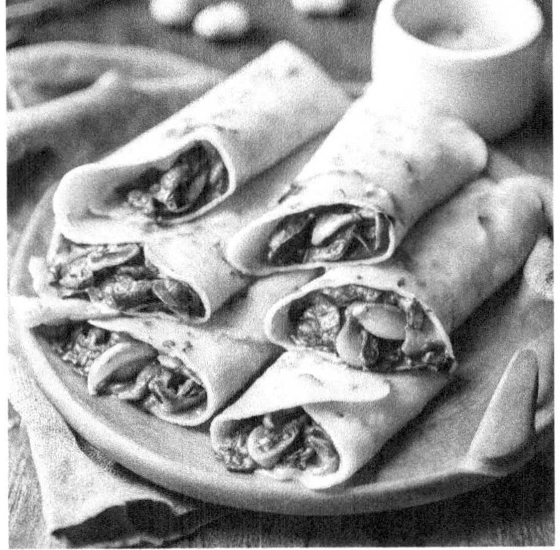

7. Quinoa and Chia Porridge

Ingredients:

- 1 cup quinoa, rinsed
- 2 cups almond milk (or any plant-based milk)
- 1 tablespoon chia seeds
- 1 teaspoon cinnamon
- 1 tablespoon maple syrup or honey
- 1/2 teaspoon vanilla extract
- Fresh berries or sliced fruit for topping

Instructions:

1. In a saucepan, combine quinoa and almond milk. Bring to a boil over medium-high heat.
2. Reduce heat to low, cover, and simmer for about 15 minutes, or until the quinoa is tender and the liquid is absorbed.
3. Stir in chia seeds, cinnamon, maple syrup or honey, and vanilla extract.
4. Cook for an additional 5 minutes, stirring occasionally, until the porridge thickens.
5. Serve warm, topped with fresh berries or sliced fruit.

Number of Serves: 4

Nutritional Info per Serving:

- Calories: 220
- Protein: 6g
- Carbohydrates: 35g
- Fiber: 5g
- Sugars: 7g
- Fat: 6g

Cooking Time: 25 minutes

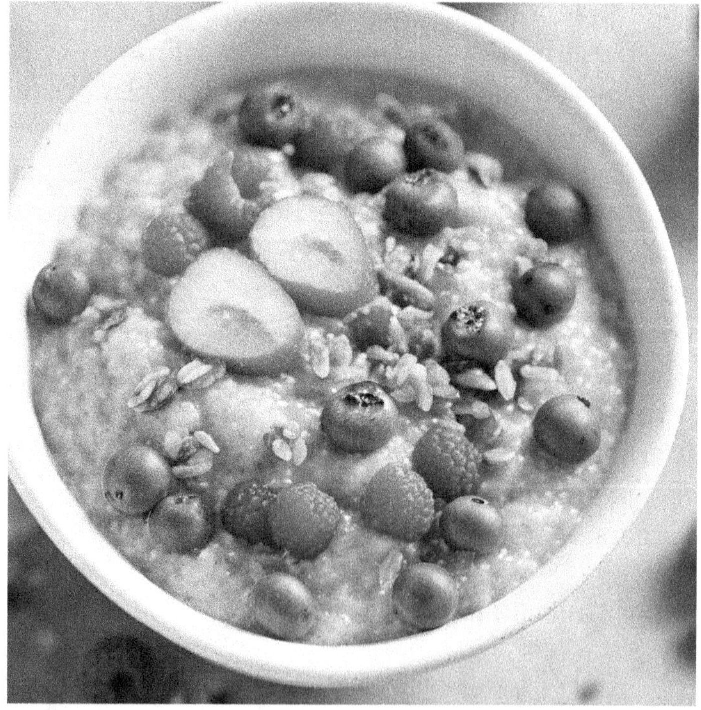

8. Fruit Salad

Ingredients:

- 1 cup strawberries, hulled and halved
- 1 cup blueberries
- 1 cup kiwi, peeled and sliced
- 1 cup mango, peeled and diced
- 1 tablespoon fresh lime juice
- 1 tablespoon honey or maple syrup (optional)
- Fresh mint leaves for garnish (optional)

Instructions:

1. In a large bowl, combine strawberries, blueberries, kiwi, and mango.
2. Drizzle with fresh lime juice and honey or maple syrup, if using.
3. Gently toss to combine.
4. Garnish with fresh mint leaves, if desired.
5. Serve immediately or chill in the refrigerator until ready to serve.

Number of Serves: 4

Nutritional Info per Serving:

- Calories: 90
- Protein: 1g
- Carbohydrates: 22g
- Fiber: 4g
- Sugars: 16g
- Fat: 0g

Cooking Time: 10 minutes

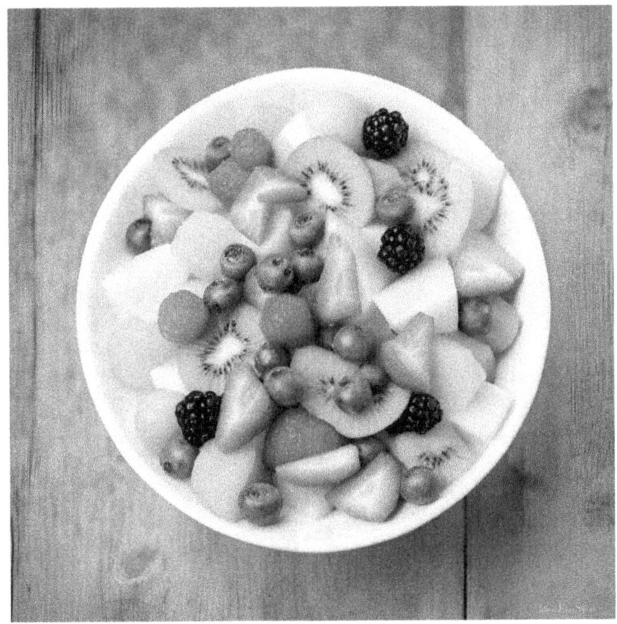

9. Amaranth Porridge

Ingredients:

- 1 cup amaranth
- 2 cups water
- 1 cup almond milk (or any plant-based milk)
- 1 tablespoon maple syrup or honey
- 1 teaspoon cinnamon
- 1/2 teaspoon vanilla extract
- Fresh fruit for topping (e.g., berries, banana slices)
- 1 tablespoon chopped nuts (optional)

Instructions:

1. In a saucepan, combine amaranth and water. Bring to a boil over medium-high heat.
2. Reduce heat to low, cover, and simmer for about 20 minutes, or until the amaranth is tender and most of the water is absorbed.
3. Stir in almond milk, maple syrup or honey, cinnamon, and vanilla extract.
4. Cook for an additional 5 minutes, stirring occasionally, until the porridge thickens.
5. Serve warm, topped with fresh fruit and chopped nuts, if desired.

Number of Serves: 4

Nutritional Info per Serving:

- Calories: 200
- Protein: 5g
- Carbohydrates: 38g
- Fiber: 4g
- Sugars: 8g
- Fat: 4g

Cooking Time: 30 minutes

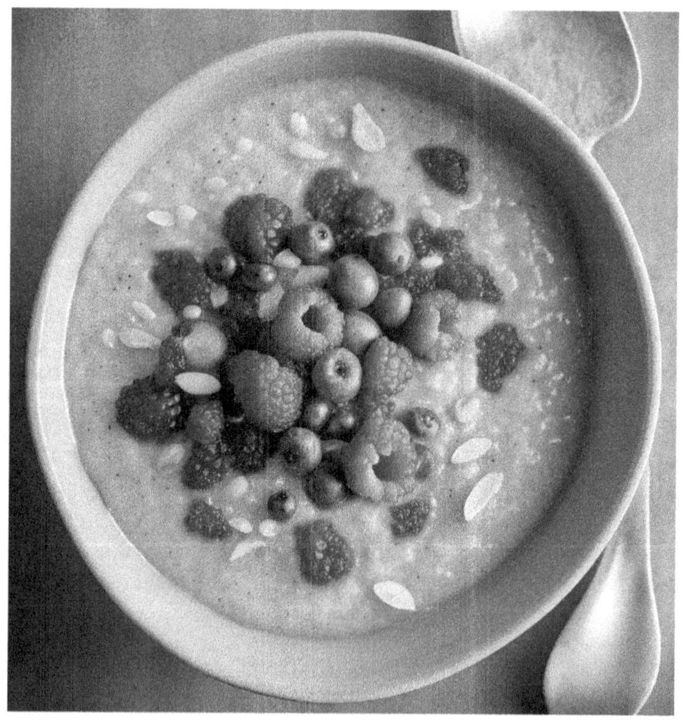

9. Pea Protein Shake

Ingredients:

- 1 cup unsweetened almond milk (or any plant-based milk)
- 1 scoop pea protein powder
- 1/2 banana
- 1/2 cup frozen berries (blueberries, strawberries, or raspberries)
- 1 tablespoon chia seeds
- 1 teaspoon vanilla extract
- 1 tablespoon almond butter (optional)

Instructions:

1. Add all ingredients to a blender.
2. Blend until smooth and creamy.
3. Pour into a glass and serve immediately.

Number of Serves: 1

Nutritional Info per Serving:

- Calories: 250
- Protein: 25g
- Carbohydrates: 25g
- Fiber: 8g
- Sugars: 10g
- Fat: 8g

Cooking Time: 5 minutes

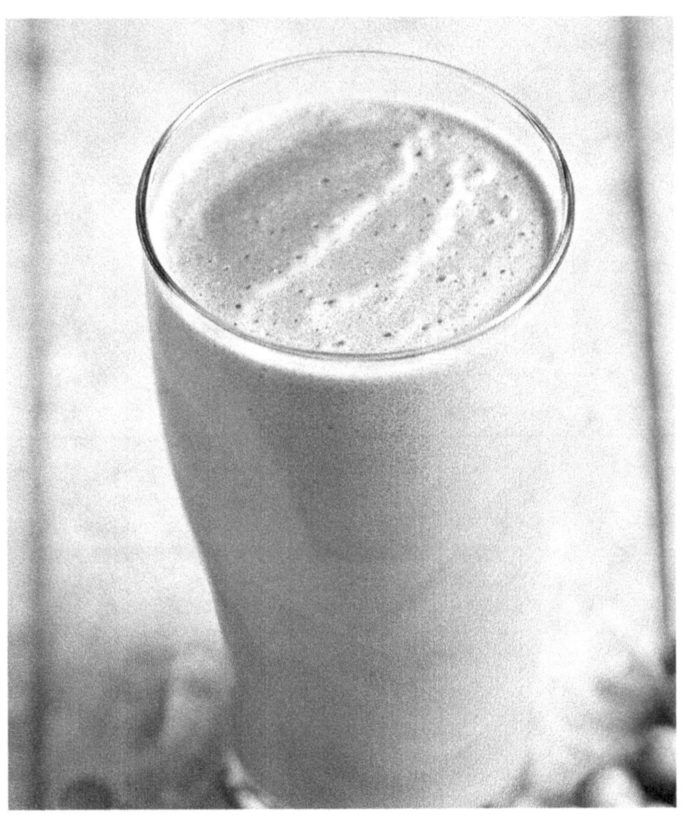

10. Almond Butter and Pear Toast

Ingredients:

- 2 slices whole-grain bread
- 2 tablespoons almond butter
- 1 ripe pear, thinly sliced
- 1 teaspoon honey or maple syrup (optional)
- 1/4 teaspoon ground cinnamon

Instructions:

1. Toast the whole-grain bread slices to your desired level of crispiness.
2. Spread 1 tablespoon of almond butter on each slice of toast.
3. Arrange the pear slices evenly on top of the almond butter.
4. Drizzle with honey or maple syrup, if using.
5. Sprinkle with ground cinnamon.
6. Serve immediately.

Number of Serves: 1

Nutritional Info per Serving:

- Calories: 320
- Protein: 10g
- Carbohydrates: 50g
- Fiber: 8g
- Sugars: 18g
- Fat: 12g

Cooking Time: 5 minutes

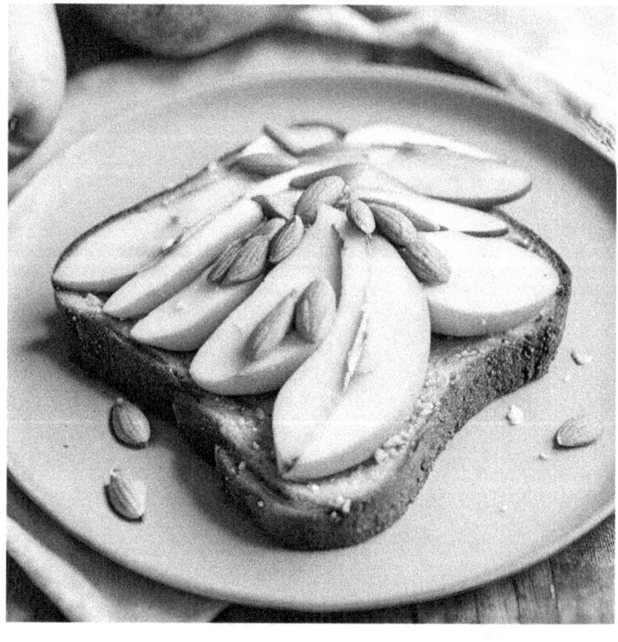

11. Flaxseed Porridge

Ingredients:

- 1/4 cup ground flaxseed
- 1 cup unsweetened almond milk (or any plant-based milk)
- 1/2 teaspoon ground cinnamon
- 1 tablespoon maple syrup or honey
- Fresh fruit for topping (e.g., berries, banana slices)
- 1 tablespoon chopped nuts (optional)

Instructions:

1. In a small saucepan, combine ground flaxseed, almond milk, and ground cinnamon.
2. Cook over medium heat, stirring frequently, until the mixture thickens, about 3-5 minutes.
3. Remove from heat and stir in maple syrup or honey.
4. Serve warm, topped with fresh fruit and chopped nuts, if desired.

Number of Serves: 1

Nutritional Info per Serving:

- Calories: 250
- Protein: 8g
- Carbohydrates: 24g
- Fiber: 12g
- Sugars: 12g
- Fat: 14g

Cooking Time: 10 minutes

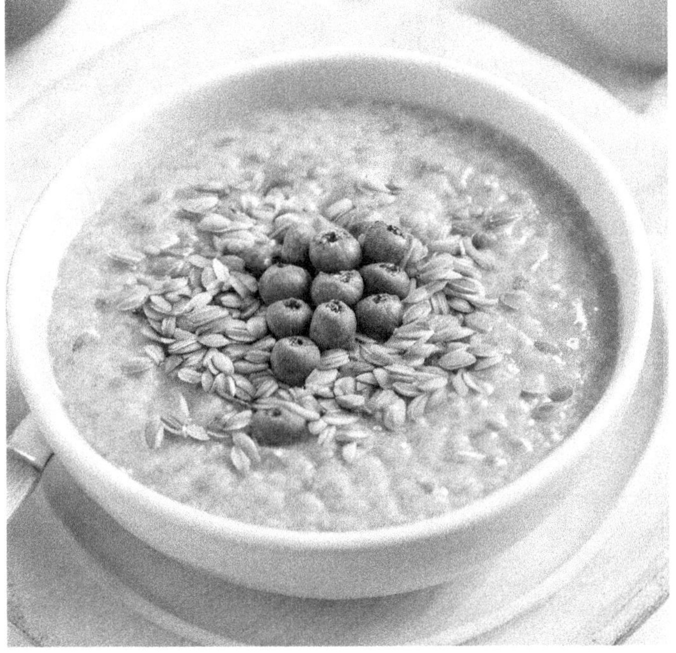

12. Roasted Beetroot Salad

Ingredients:

- 2 medium beetroots, peeled and diced
- 1 tablespoon olive oil
- 1 cup baby spinach
- 1/4 cup walnuts, chopped
- 1/4 cup feta cheese, crumbled (optional)
- 2 tablespoons balsamic vinegar
- 1 teaspoon honey or maple syrup

Instructions:

1. Preheat your oven to 400°F (200°C).
2. Toss the diced beetroots with olive oil and spread them on a baking sheet.
3. Roast in the preheated oven for 25-30 minutes, or until tender.
4. In a large bowl, combine roasted beetroots, baby spinach, walnuts, and feta cheese if using.
5. In a small bowl, whisk together balsamic vinegar and honey or maple syrup.
6. Drizzle the dressing over the salad and toss to combine.
7. Serve immediately.

Number of Serves: 2

Nutritional Info per Serving:

- Calories: 220
- Protein: 5g
- Carbohydrates: 18g
- Fiber: 6g
- Sugars: 10g
- Fat: 14g

Cooking Time: 30 minutes

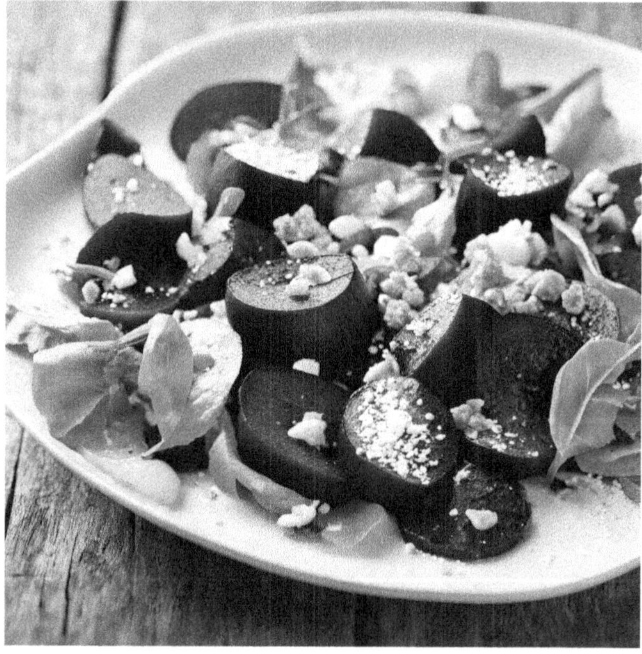

13. Zucchini Muffins

Ingredients:

- 1 cup whole wheat flour
- 1/2 cup almond flour
- 1 teaspoon baking powder
- 1/2 teaspoon baking soda
- 1 teaspoon ground cinnamon
- 1/2 teaspoon ground nutmeg
- 1/4 cup honey or maple syrup
- 1/4 cup unsweetened applesauce
- 2 large eggs
- 1/4 cup olive oil
- 1 teaspoon vanilla extract
- 1 cup grated zucchini
- 1/2 cup chopped walnuts (optional)

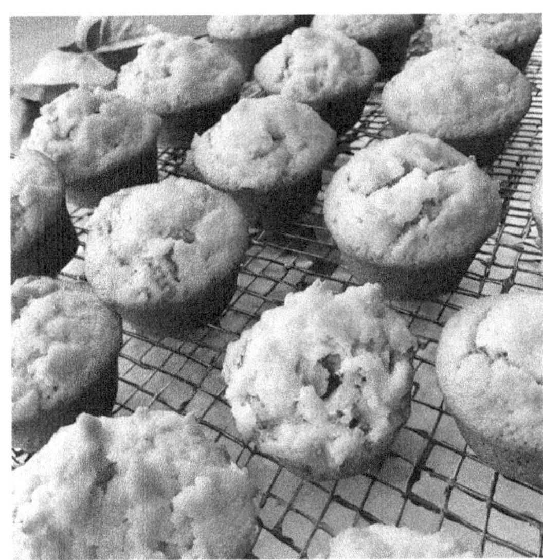

Instructions:

1. Preheat your oven to 350°F (175°C) and line a muffin tin with paper liners or grease it lightly.
2. In a large bowl, whisk together whole wheat flour, almond flour, baking powder, baking soda, ground cinnamon, and ground nutmeg.
3. In another bowl, whisk together honey or maple syrup, applesauce, eggs, olive oil, and vanilla extract.
4. Add the wet ingredients to the dry ingredients and stir until just combined.
5. Fold in the grated zucchini and walnuts, if using.
6. Divide the batter evenly among the muffin cups.
7. Bake for 20-25 minutes, or until a toothpick inserted into the center comes out clean.
8. Allow the muffins to cool in the tin for 5 minutes before transferring to a wire rack to cool completely.

Number of Serves: 12 muffins

Nutritional Info per Serving:

- Calories: 160
- Protein: 4g
- Carbohydrates: 18g
- Fiber: 3g
- Sugars: 7g
- Fat: 9g

Cooking Time: 30 minutes

14. Kale Smoothie
Ingredients:
- 1 cup unsweetened almond milk (or any plant-based milk)
- 1 cup fresh kale, stems removed
- 1/2 banana
- 1/2 cup frozen pineapple chunks
- 1 tablespoon chia seeds
- 1 teaspoon fresh lemon juice
- 1 teaspoon honey or maple syrup (optional)

Instructions:
1. Add all ingredients to a blender.
2. Blend until smooth and creamy.
3. Pour into a glass and serve immediately.

Number of Serves: 1
Nutritional Info per Serving:
- Calories: 180
- Protein: 5g
- Carbohydrates: 30g
- Fiber: 7g
- Sugars: 15g
- Fat: 5g

Cooking Time: 5 minutes

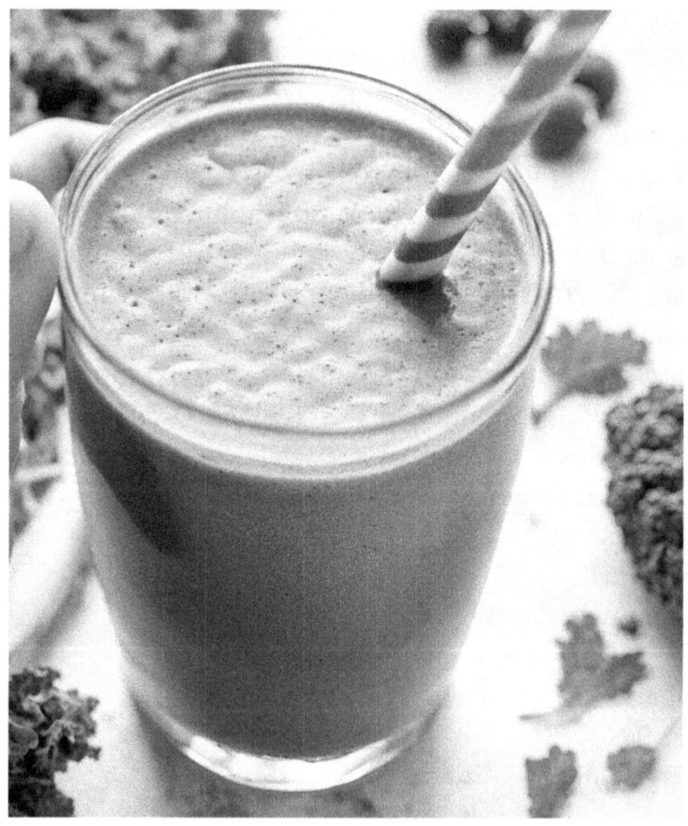

15. Mixed Berry Salad

Ingredients:

- 1 cup strawberries, hulled and sliced
- 1 cup blueberries
- 1 cup raspberries
- 1 cup blackberries
- 1 tablespoon fresh lemon juice
- 1 tablespoon honey or maple syrup (optional)
- Fresh mint leaves for garnish (optional)

Instructions:

1. In a large bowl, combine strawberries, blueberries, raspberries, and blackberries.
2. Drizzle with fresh lemon juice and honey or maple syrup, if using.
3. Gently toss to combine.
4. Garnish with fresh mint leaves, if desired.
5. Serve immediately or chill in the refrigerator until ready to serve.

Number of Serves: 4

Nutritional Info per Serving:

- Calories: 70
- Protein: 1g
- Carbohydrates: 18g
- Fiber: 6g
- Sugars: 10g
- Fat: 0g

Cooking Time: 10 minutes

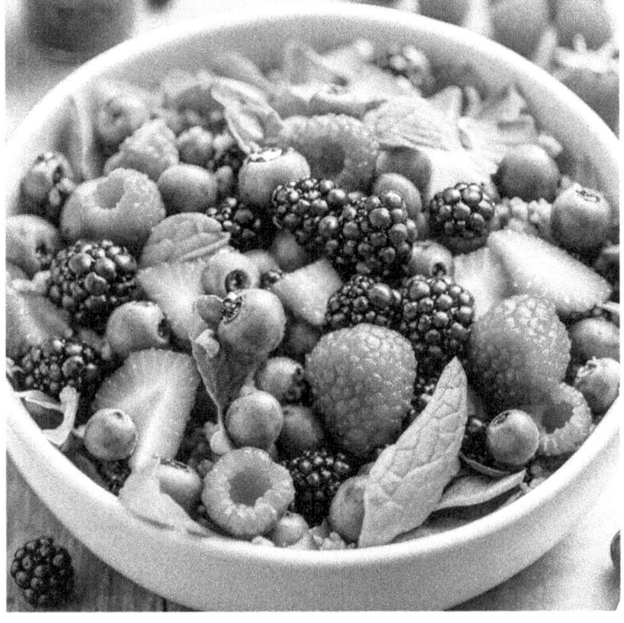

16. Sautéed Tempeh

Ingredients:

- 1 block (8 ounces) tempeh, sliced into thin strips
- 2 tablespoons olive oil
- 2 tablespoons tamari or low-sodium soy sauce
- 1 tablespoon apple cider vinegar
- 1 clove garlic, minced
- 1 teaspoon fresh ginger, grated

Instructions:

1. In a bowl, mix tamari or soy sauce, apple cider vinegar, garlic, and ginger.
2. Add the sliced tempeh to the bowl and let it marinate for at least 15 minutes.
3. Heat olive oil in a skillet over medium heat.
4. Add the marinated tempeh strips and sauté for 5-7 minutes, until golden brown and crispy.
5. Serve immediately.

Number of Serves: 4

Nutritional Info per Serving:

- Calories: 150
- Protein: 12g
- Carbohydrates: 8g
- Fiber: 3g
- Sugars: 1g
- Fat: 9g

Cooking Time: 20 minutes (including marinating time)

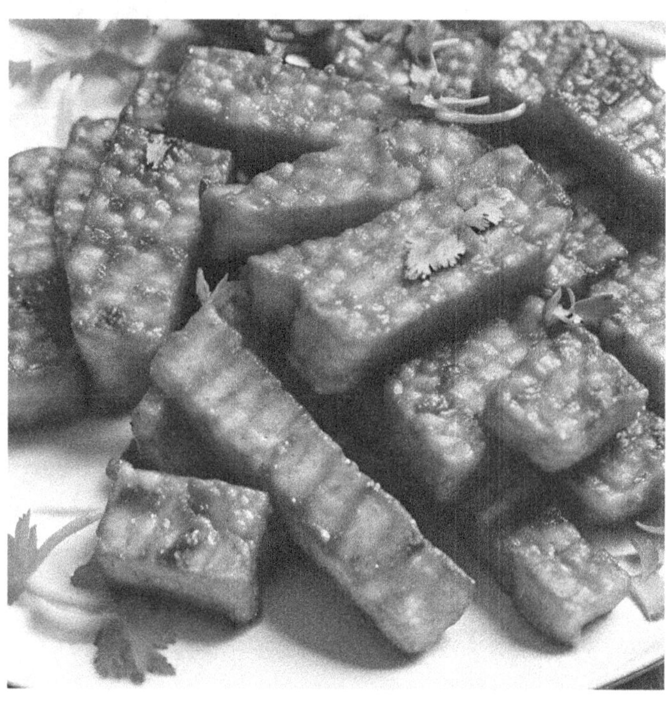

17. Mango and Spinach Smoothie

Ingredients:

- 1 cup unsweetened almond milk (or any plant-based milk)
- 1 cup fresh spinach
- 1 cup frozen mango chunks
- 1/2 banana
- 1 tablespoon chia seeds
- 1 teaspoon fresh lime juice

Instructions:

1. Add all ingredients to a blender.
2. Blend until smooth and creamy.
3. Pour into a glass and serve immediately.

Number of Serves: 1

Nutritional Info per Serving:

- Calories: 200
- Protein: 4g
- Carbohydrates: 40g
- Fiber: 7g
- Sugars: 30g
- Fat: 5g

Cooking Time: 5 minutes

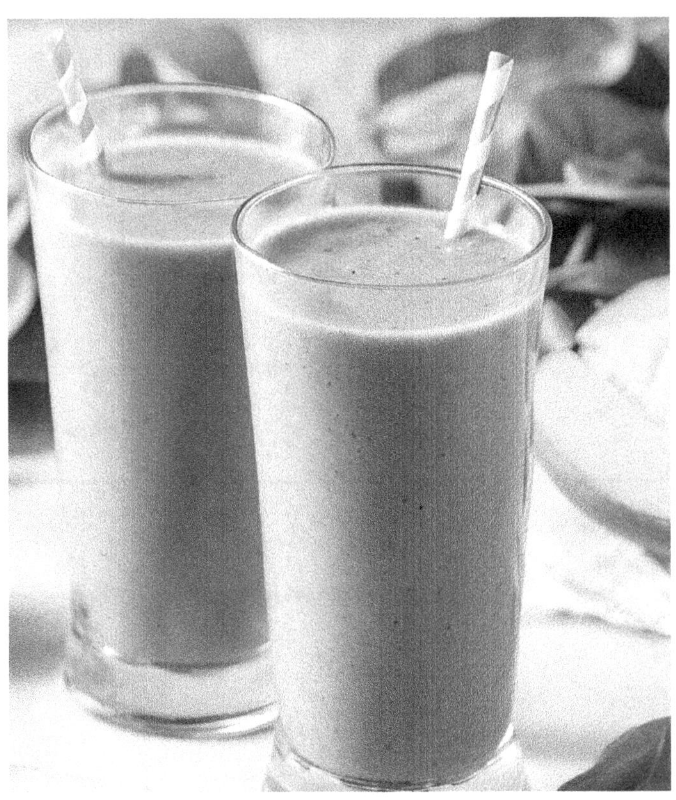

18. Pumpkin Porridge

Ingredients:

- 1 cup rolled oats
- 2 cups unsweetened almond milk (or any plant-based milk)
- 1/2 cup pumpkin puree
- 1 tablespoon maple syrup or honey
- 1 teaspoon ground cinnamon
- 1/2 teaspoon ground nutmeg
- 1/4 teaspoon ground ginger
- 1/4 cup chopped walnuts (optional)

Instructions:

1. In a saucepan, combine rolled oats and almond milk. Bring to a boil over medium-high heat.
2. Reduce heat to low and stir in pumpkin puree, maple syrup or honey, cinnamon, nutmeg, and ginger.
3. Cook for about 5 minutes, stirring occasionally, until the porridge is thick and creamy.
4. Serve warm, topped with chopped walnuts if desired.

Number of Serves: 4

Nutritional Info per Serving:

- Calories: 220
- Protein: 6g
- Carbohydrates: 38g
- Fiber: 7g
- Sugars: 10g
- Fat: 6g

Cooking Time: 10 minutes

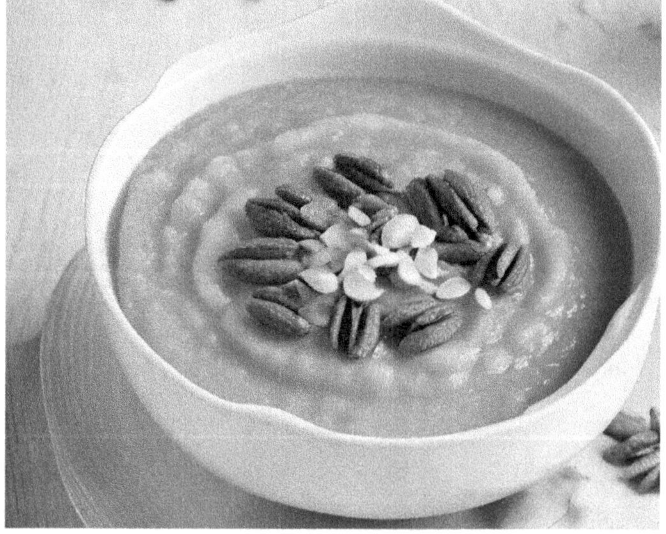

19. Banana Almond Smoothie
Ingredients:
- 1 cup unsweetened almond milk (or any plant-based milk)
- 1 banana
- 1 tablespoon almond butter
- 1 tablespoon chia seeds
- 1/2 teaspoon vanilla extract
- 1/2 teaspoon ground cinnamon

Instructions:
1. Add all ingredients to a blender.
2. Blend until smooth and creamy.
3. Pour into a glass and serve immediately.

Number of Serves: 1
Nutritional Info per Serving:
- Calories: 250
- Protein: 6g
- Carbohydrates: 40g
- Fiber: 8g
- Sugars: 18g
- Fat: 10g

Cooking Time: 5 minutes

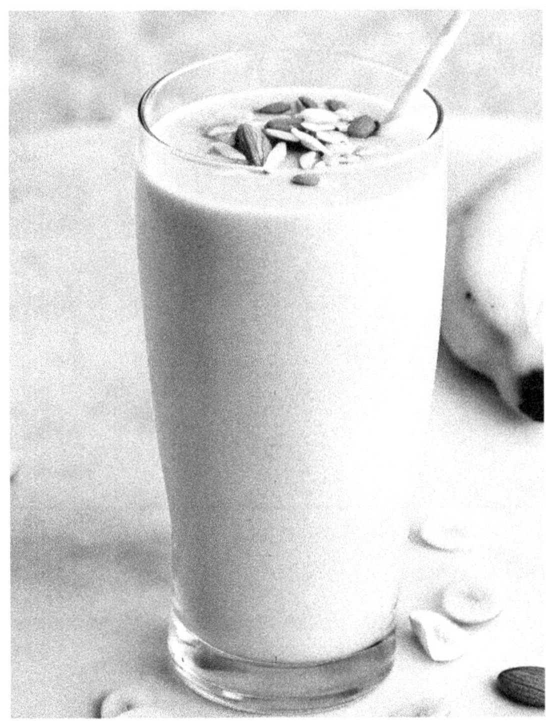

20. Savory Quinoa Bowl

Ingredients:

- 1 cup quinoa, rinsed
- 2 cups water
- 1 tablespoon olive oil
- 1 cup cherry tomatoes, halved
- 1 avocado, diced
- 1/2 cup cucumber, diced
- 1/4 cup red onion, finely chopped
- 1/4 cup fresh cilantro, chopped
- 1 tablespoon fresh lemon juice

Instructions:

1. In a saucepan, combine quinoa and water. Bring to a boil over medium-high heat.
2. Reduce heat to low, cover, and simmer for about 15 minutes, or until the quinoa is tender and the water is absorbed.
3. In a large bowl, combine cooked quinoa, cherry tomatoes, avocado, cucumber, red onion, and fresh cilantro.
4. Drizzle with olive oil and fresh lemon juice, and toss to combine.
5. Serve immediately.

Number of Serves: 4

Nutritional Info per Serving:

- Calories: 280
- Protein: 7g
- Carbohydrates: 35g
- Fiber: 8g
- Sugars: 5g
- Fat: 14g

Cooking Time: 20 minutes

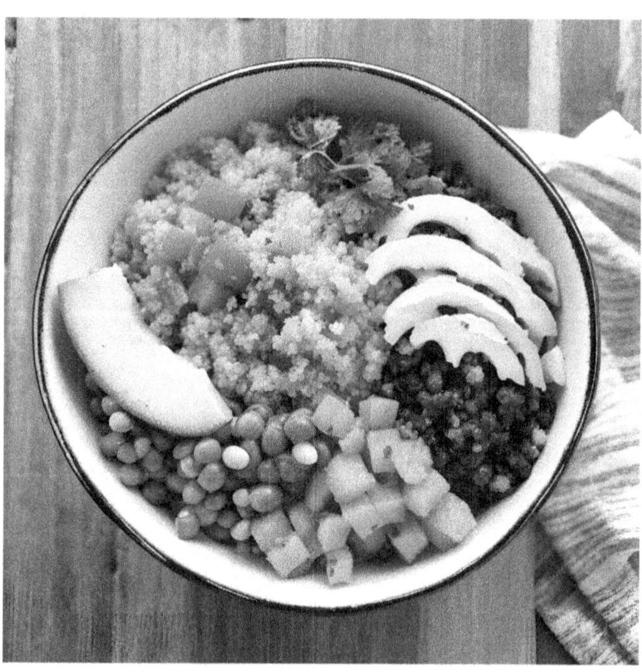

21. Turmeric Latte

Ingredients:

- 1 cup unsweetened almond milk (or any plant-based milk)
- 1 teaspoon ground turmeric
- 1/2 teaspoon ground cinnamon
- 1/4 teaspoon ground ginger
- 1/4 teaspoon vanilla extract
- 1 tablespoon honey or maple syrup (optional)
- Pinch of black pepper (to enhance absorption of turmeric)

Instructions:

1. In a small saucepan, combine almond milk, turmeric, cinnamon, ginger, and black pepper.
2. Heat over medium heat, stirring constantly, until the mixture is hot but not boiling.
3. Remove from heat and stir in vanilla extract and honey or maple syrup if using.
4. Use a whisk or a milk frother to froth the mixture until it becomes creamy.
5. Pour into a mug and serve immediately.

Number of Serves: 1

Nutritional Info per Serving:

- Calories: 80
- Protein: 1g
- Carbohydrates: 12g
- Fiber: 2g
- Sugars: 8g
- Fat: 3g

Cooking Time: 5 minutes

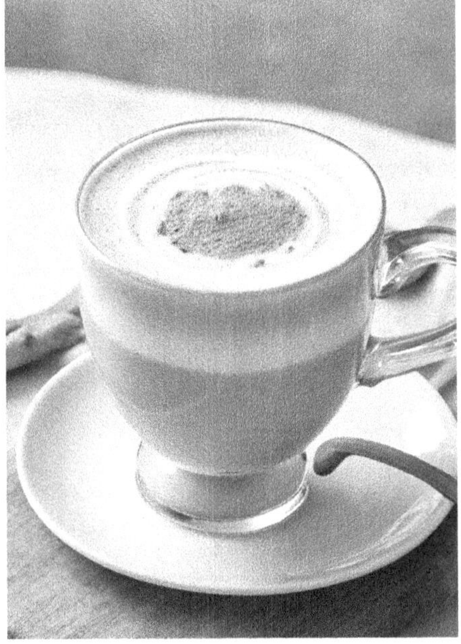

22. Buckwheat Pancakes

Ingredients:

- 1 cup buckwheat flour
- 1 teaspoon baking powder
- 1/2 teaspoon ground cinnamon
- 1 cup unsweetened almond milk (or any plant-based milk)
- 1 large egg
- 2 tablespoons maple syrup or honey
- 1 teaspoon vanilla extract
- 1 tablespoon olive oil or coconut oil for cooking

Instructions:

1. In a large bowl, whisk together buckwheat flour, baking powder, and ground cinnamon.
2. In another bowl, whisk together almond milk, egg, maple syrup or honey, and vanilla extract.
3. Pour the wet ingredients into the dry ingredients and stir until just combined.
4. Heat a non-stick skillet or griddle over medium heat and lightly coat with olive oil or coconut oil.
5. Pour 1/4 cup of batter onto the skillet for each pancake. Cook until bubbles form on the surface, about 2-3 minutes, then flip and cook for another 1-2 minutes until golden brown.
6. Repeat with the remaining batter.
7. Serve warm with additional maple syrup, fresh fruit, or your favorite toppings.

Number of Serves: 4 (makes about 8 pancakes)

Nutritional Info per Serving (2 pancakes):

- Calories: 200
- Protein: 6g
- Carbohydrates: 35g
- Fiber: 4g
- Sugars: 7g
- Fat: 5g

Cooking Time: 20 minutes

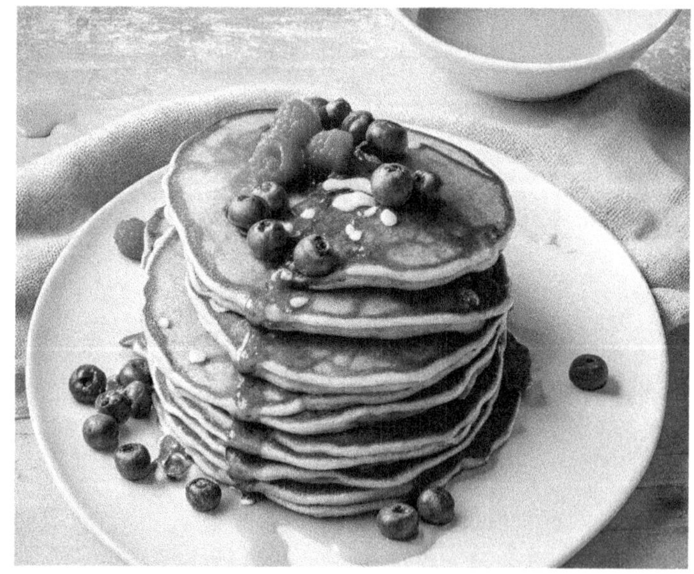

23. Oatmeal with Berries

Ingredients:

- 1 cup rolled oats
- 2 cups water or unsweetened almond milk (or any plant-based milk)
- 1 tablespoon chia seeds
- 1 teaspoon ground cinnamon
- 1 tablespoon honey or maple syrup
- 1 cup mixed berries (blueberries, strawberries, raspberries)
- 1/4 cup chopped nuts (optional)

Instructions:

1. In a saucepan, combine rolled oats and water or almond milk. Bring to a boil over medium-high heat.
2. Reduce heat to low and stir in chia seeds and ground cinnamon.
3. Cook for about 5 minutes, stirring occasionally, until the oats are tender and the porridge is creamy.
4. Remove from heat and stir in honey or maple syrup.
5. Serve warm, topped with mixed berries and chopped nuts if desired.

Number of Serves: 2

Nutritional Info per Serving:

- Calories: 280
- Protein: 6g
- Carbohydrates: 45g
- Fiber: 8g
- Sugars: 15g
- Fat: 8g

Cooking Time: 10 minutes

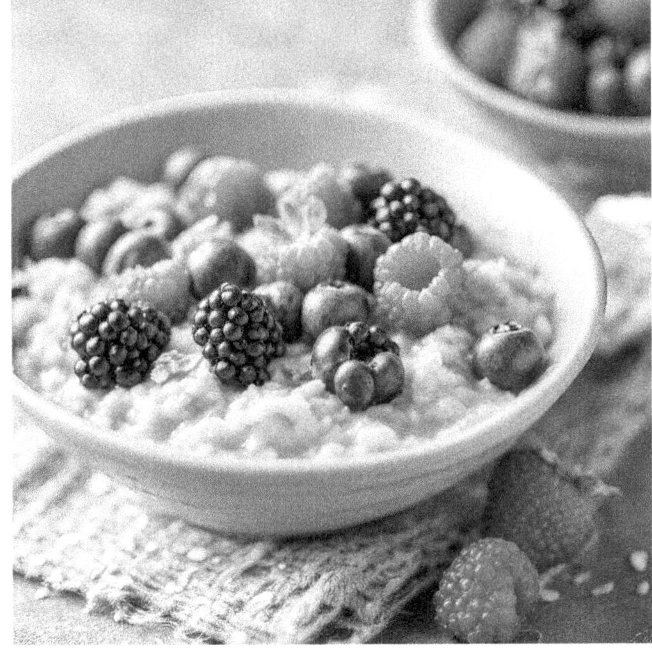

Poultry Recipes

1. Grilled Chicken with Avocado Salsa
Ingredients:
- For the chicken:
    - 4 boneless, skinless chicken breasts
    - 2 tablespoons olive oil
    - 1 tablespoon lime juice
    - 1 teaspoon ground cumin
    - 1 teaspoon garlic powder
- For the avocado salsa:
    - 2 ripe avocados, diced
    - 1 cup cherry tomatoes, halved
    - 1/4 cup red onion, finely chopped
    - 1/4 cup fresh cilantro, chopped
    - 1 tablespoon lime juice

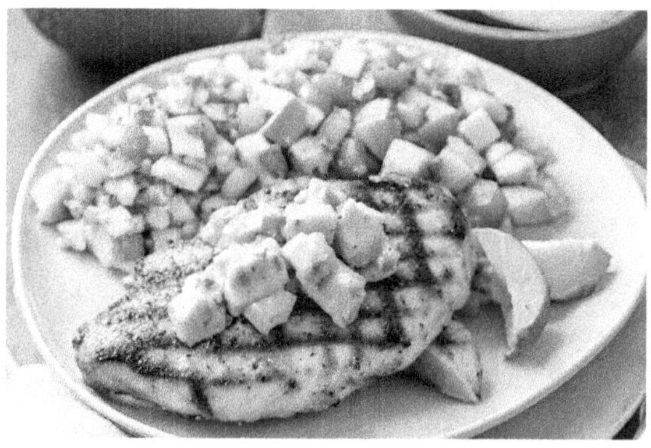

Instructions:
1. Marinate the chicken:
    - In a small bowl, mix olive oil, lime juice, ground cumin, and garlic powder.
    - Rub the mixture over the chicken breasts and let marinate for at least 30 minutes.
2. Prepare the salsa:
    - In a medium bowl, combine diced avocados, cherry tomatoes, red onion, cilantro, and lime juice. Gently mix and set aside.
3. Grill the chicken:
    - Preheat the grill to medium-high heat.
    - Grill the chicken breasts for 6-7 minutes per side, or until fully cooked and juices run clear.
4. Serve:
    - Plate the grilled chicken and top with avocado salsa.
    - Serve immediately.

Number of Serves: 4
Nutritional Info per Serving:
- Calories: 350   Protein: 30g   Carbohydrates: 12g
- Fiber: 7g   Sugars: 2g   Fat: 20g

Cooking Time: 45 minutes (including marinating time)

2. Turmeric Chicken Soup

Ingredients:

- 1 tablespoon olive oil
- 1 onion, chopped
- 2 cloves garlic, minced
- 1 teaspoon ground turmeric
- 1 teaspoon ground ginger
- 4 boneless, skinless chicken thighs, cut into bite-sized pieces
- 6 cups low-sodium chicken broth
- 2 carrots, sliced
- 2 celery stalks, sliced
- 1 cup chopped kale
- 1/2 cup quinoa, rinsed
- Juice of 1 lemon

Instructions:

1. Sauté the aromatics:
   - Heat olive oil in a large pot over medium heat.
   - Add onion and garlic and cook until softened, about 5 minutes.
   - Stir in turmeric and ginger.
2. Cook the chicken:
   - Add chicken thighs to the pot and cook until browned, about 5 minutes.
3. Simmer the soup:
   - Pour in the chicken broth, carrots, celery, and quinoa.
   - Bring to a boil, then reduce heat and simmer for 20 minutes, or until the quinoa and vegetables are tender.
4. Finish and serve:
   - Stir in kale and cook for an additional 5 minutes.
   - Add lemon juice just before serving.
   - Serve hot.

Number of Serves: 6

Nutritional Info per Serving:

- Calories: 220
- Protein: 18g
- Carbohydrates: 20g
- Fiber: 4g
- Sugars: 3g
- Fat: 8g

Cooking Time: 40 minutes

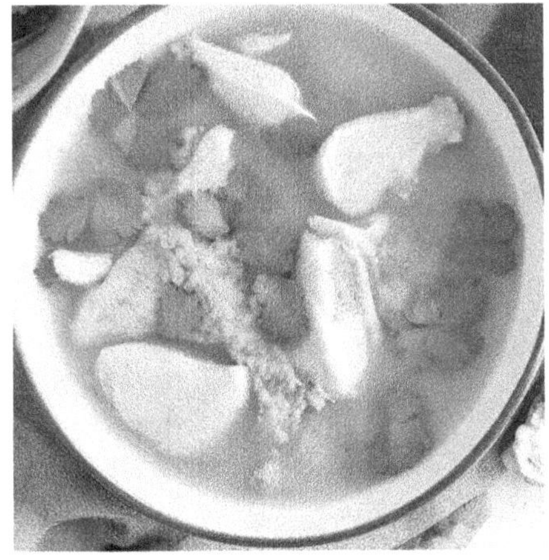

3. Baked Lemon and Herb Chicken

Ingredients:

- 4 boneless, skinless chicken breasts
- 3 tablespoons olive oil
- 2 tablespoons fresh lemon juice
- 2 cloves garlic, minced
- 1 tablespoon fresh thyme, chopped
- 1 tablespoon fresh rosemary, chopped
- 1 teaspoon lemon zest

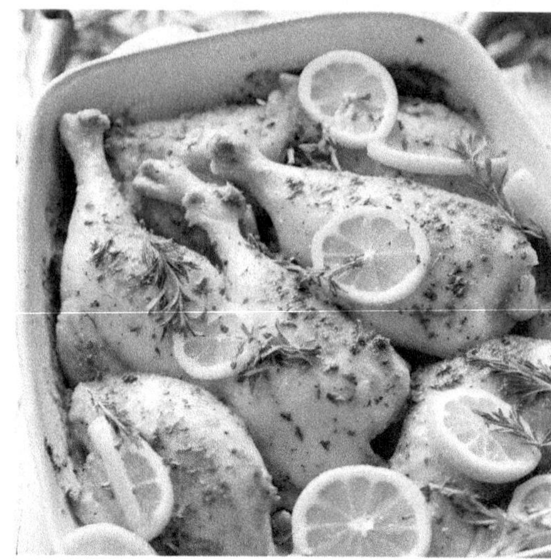

Instructions:

1. Preheat oven:
   - Preheat your oven to 375°F (190°C).
2. Prepare the marinade:
   - In a small bowl, combine olive oil, lemon juice, garlic, thyme, rosemary, and lemon zest.
3. Marinate the chicken:
   - Place the chicken breasts in a baking dish and pour the marinade over them, ensuring they are well coated.
   - Let marinate for at least 15 minutes.
4. Bake the chicken:
   - Bake in the preheated oven for 25-30 minutes, or until the chicken is cooked through and juices run clear.
5. Serve:
   - Serve the baked chicken with your favorite side dishes.

Number of Serves: 4

Nutritional Info per Serving:

- Calories: 280
- Protein: 28g
- Carbohydrates: 2g
- Fiber: 1g
- Sugars: 0g
- Fat: 18g

Cooking Time: 45 minutes (including marinating time)

4. Chicken and Quinoa Salad

Ingredients:

- 1 cup quinoa, rinsed
- 2 cups water
- 2 boneless, skinless chicken breasts
- 2 tablespoons olive oil, divided
- 1 cup cherry tomatoes, halved
- 1/2 cup cucumber, diced
- 1/4 cup red onion, finely chopped
- 1/4 cup fresh parsley, chopped
- 2 tablespoons lemon juice
- 1 tablespoon balsamic vinegar

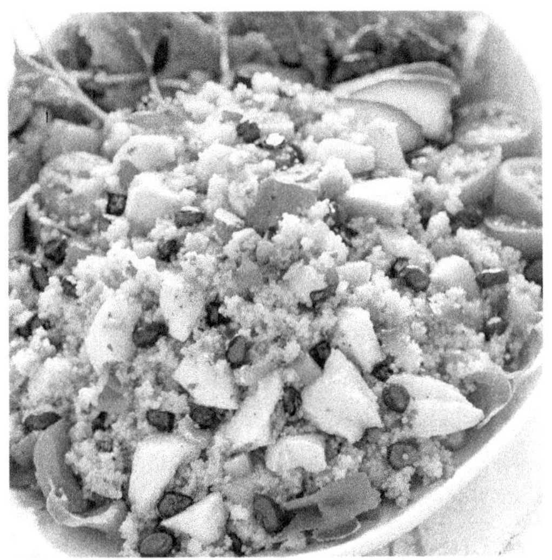

Instructions:

1. Cook the quinoa:
   - In a saucepan, bring quinoa and water to a boil.
   - Reduce heat, cover, and simmer for 15 minutes, or until the quinoa is tender and water is absorbed. Set aside to cool.
2. Cook the chicken:
   - Heat 1 tablespoon of olive oil in a skillet over medium heat.
   - Add chicken breasts and cook for about 6-7 minutes per side, or until fully cooked. Let cool and then dice.
3. Prepare the salad:
   - In a large bowl, combine cooked quinoa, diced chicken, cherry tomatoes, cucumber, red onion, and parsley.
4. Make the dressing:
   - In a small bowl, whisk together lemon juice, balsamic vinegar, and the remaining 1 tablespoon of olive oil.
5. Combine and serve:
   - Pour the dressing over the salad and toss to combine.
   - Serve immediately or chill in the refrigerator until ready to serve.

Number of Serves: 4

Nutritional Info per Serving:

- Calories: 350
- Protein: 28g
- Carbohydrates: 30g
- Fiber: 5g
- Sugars: 4g
- Fat: 14g

Cooking Time: 30 minutes

5. Garlic Ginger Chicken Stir-Fry

Ingredients:

- 1 lb (450g) boneless, skinless chicken breast, sliced into thin strips
- 2 tablespoons olive oil
- 3 cloves garlic, minced
- 1 tablespoon fresh ginger, minced
- 1 red bell pepper, sliced
- 1 cup broccoli florets
- 1 carrot, thinly sliced
- 1/4 cup low-sodium soy sauce or tamari
- 2 tablespoons honey or maple syrup
- 1 tablespoon rice vinegar
- 1 teaspoon sesame oil
- 1 tablespoon sesame seeds (optional)

Instructions:

1. Heat olive oil in a large skillet or wok over medium-high heat.
2. Add the chicken strips and cook until no longer pink, about 5-7 minutes. Remove and set aside.
3. In the same skillet, add garlic and ginger, cooking for 1-2 minutes until fragrant.
4. Add red bell pepper, broccoli, and carrot. Stir-fry for about 5 minutes until vegetables are tender-crisp.
5. In a small bowl, mix soy sauce or tamari, honey or maple syrup, rice vinegar, and sesame oil.
6. Return the chicken to the skillet and pour the sauce over. Stir well to combine and cook for another 2-3 minutes.
7. Garnish with sesame seeds if desired. Serve immediately.

Number of Serves: 4

Nutritional Info per Serving:

- Calories: 260
- Protein: 28g
- Carbohydrates: 18g
- Fiber: 3g
- Sugars: 10g
- Fat: 10g

Cooking Time: 20 minutes

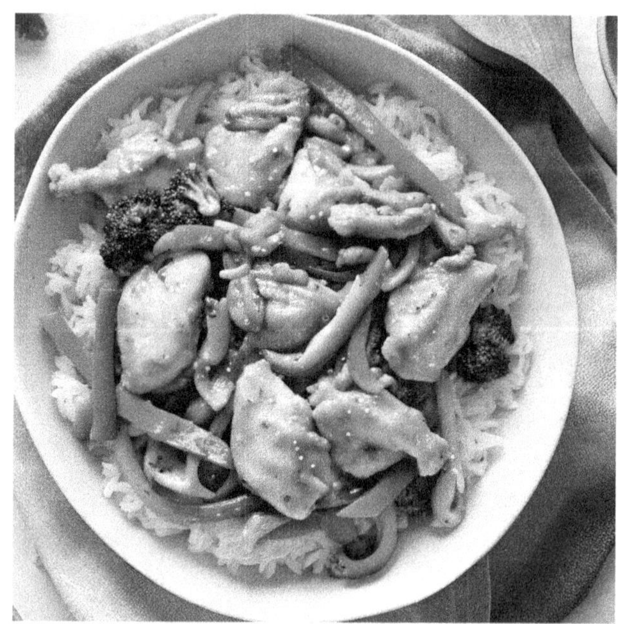

6. Slow Cooker Chicken Cacciatore

Ingredients:

- 4 boneless, skinless chicken thighs
- 1 onion, chopped
- 3 cloves garlic, minced
- 1 red bell pepper, sliced
- 1 yellow bell pepper, sliced
- 1 (14.5 oz) can diced tomatoes
- 1/4 cup tomato paste
- 1/2 cup low-sodium chicken broth
- 1 teaspoon dried oregano
- 1 teaspoon dried basil
- 1/2 teaspoon dried thyme
- 1/4 cup black olives, sliced (optional)

Instructions:

1. Place the chicken thighs in the slow cooker.
2. Add onion, garlic, red and yellow bell peppers, diced tomatoes, tomato paste, chicken broth, oregano, basil, and thyme.
3. Cover and cook on low for 6-8 hours or on high for 3-4 hours until the chicken is tender and fully cooked.
4. Add sliced olives during the last 30 minutes of cooking if desired.
5. Serve hot over whole-grain pasta or with a side of vegetables.

Number of Serves: 4

Nutritional Info per Serving:

- Calories: 220
- Protein: 24g
- Carbohydrates: 16g
- Fiber: 4g
- Sugars: 8g
- Fat: 7g

Cooking Time: 6-8 hours (slow cooker)

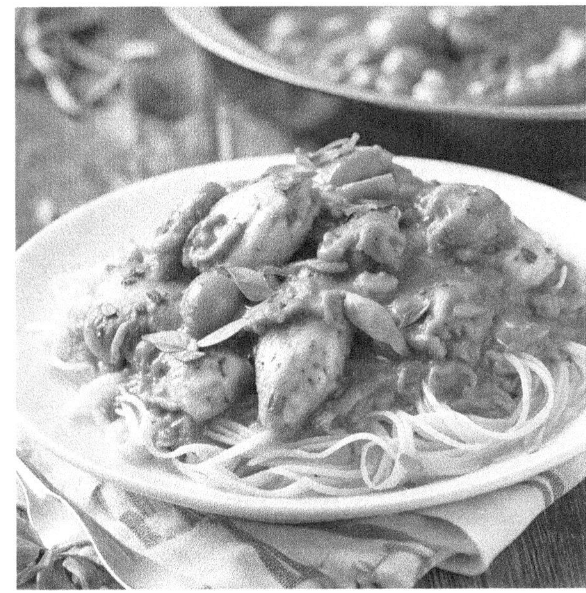

7. Moroccan Chicken Stew

Ingredients:

- 1 lb (450g) boneless, skinless chicken thighs, cut into chunks
- 2 tablespoons olive oil
- 1 onion, chopped
- 2 cloves garlic, minced
- 1 teaspoon ground cumin
- 1 teaspoon ground cinnamon
- 1 teaspoon ground ginger
- 1/2 teaspoon turmeric
- 1/4 teaspoon cayenne pepper (optional)
- 1 (14.5 oz) can diced tomatoes
- 1 cup low-sodium chicken broth
- 1 cup carrots, sliced
- 1 cup sweet potato, cubed
- 1/2 cup dried apricots, chopped
- 1/4 cup fresh cilantro, chopped

Instructions:

1. Heat olive oil in a large pot over medium heat. Add the chicken and brown on all sides, about 5 minutes. Remove and set aside.
2. In the same pot, add onion and garlic, and cook until softened, about 3-4 minutes.
3. Stir in cumin, cinnamon, ginger, turmeric, and cayenne pepper (if using).
4. Add diced tomatoes, chicken broth, carrots, sweet potato, and dried apricots.
5. Return the chicken to the pot, bring to a boil, then reduce heat and simmer for 25-30 minutes until the vegetables and chicken are tender.
6. Stir in fresh cilantro before serving.

Number of Serves: 4

Nutritional Info per Serving:

- Calories: 320
- Protein: 24g
- Carbohydrates: 35g
- Fiber: 7g
- Sugars: 16g
- Fat: 10g

Cooking Time: 45 minutes

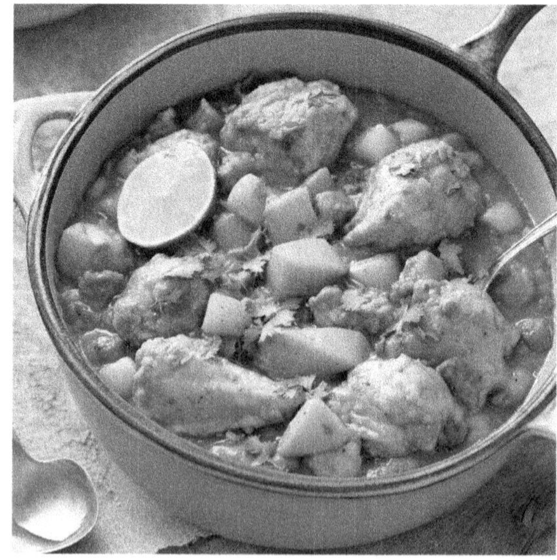

8. Apple Cider Vinegar Chicken

Ingredients:

- 4 boneless, skinless chicken breasts
- 1/4 cup apple cider vinegar
- 1/4 cup olive oil
- 2 cloves garlic, minced
- 1 tablespoon Dijon mustard
- 1 tablespoon honey or maple syrup
- 1 teaspoon dried thyme

Instructions:

1. In a small bowl, whisk together apple cider vinegar, olive oil, garlic, Dijon mustard, honey or maple syrup, and thyme.
2. Place the chicken breasts in a shallow dish and pour the marinade over them. Let marinate for at least 30 minutes, preferably 2 hours.
3. Preheat the oven to 375°F (190°C).
4. Transfer the chicken breasts to a baking dish and pour the marinade over them.
5. Bake for 25-30 minutes, or until the chicken is cooked through and juices run clear.
6. Serve immediately.

Number of Serves: 4

Nutritional Info per Serving:

- Calories: 250
- Protein: 28g
- Carbohydrates: 6g
- Fiber: 0g
- Sugars: 5g
- Fat: 12g

Cooking Time: 45 minutes (including marinating time)

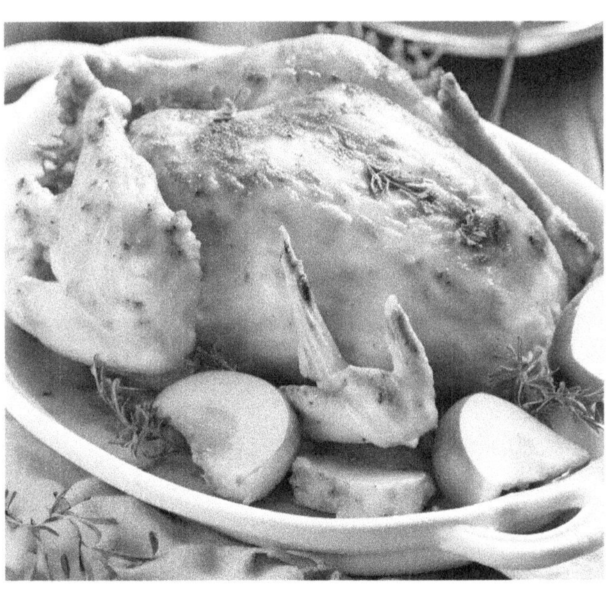

9. Spinach and Walnut Stuffed Chicken

Ingredients:

- 4 boneless, skinless chicken breasts
- 1 cup fresh spinach, chopped
- 1/2 cup walnuts, chopped
- 1/4 cup feta cheese, crumbled
- 1 clove garlic, minced
- 2 tablespoons olive oil
- 1 tablespoon lemon juice

Instructions:

1. Preheat oven to 375°F (190°C).
2. In a bowl, combine spinach, walnuts, feta cheese, and garlic.
3. Slice a pocket into each chicken breast and stuff with the spinach mixture.
4. Secure with toothpicks if needed.
5. Place the stuffed chicken breasts in a baking dish.
6. Drizzle with olive oil and lemon juice.
7. Bake for 25-30 minutes, or until the chicken is cooked through and the filling is hot.
8. Serve immediately.

Number of Serves: 4

Nutritional Info per Serving:

- Calories: 320
- Protein: 30g
- Carbohydrates: 5g
- Fiber: 2g
- Sugars: 1g
- Fat: 20g

Cooking Time: 35 minutes

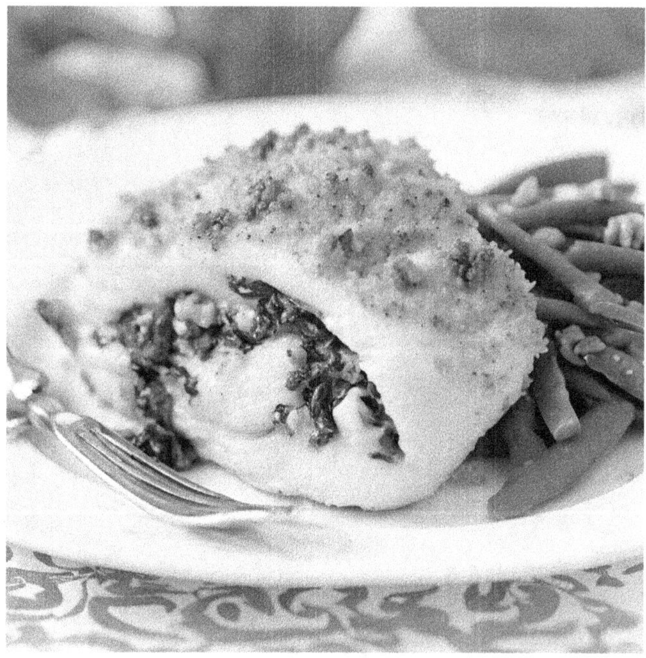

10. Paleo Chicken Tenders

Ingredients:

- 1 lb (450g) chicken tenders
- 1 cup almond flour
- 1/2 cup unsweetened shredded coconut
- 1 teaspoon paprika
- 1/2 teaspoon garlic powder
- 2 large eggs, beaten
- 2 tablespoons coconut oil (for frying)

Instructions:

1. In a shallow bowl, mix almond flour, shredded coconut, paprika, and garlic powder.
2. Dip each chicken tender into the beaten eggs, then coat with the almond flour mixture.
3. Heat coconut oil in a large skillet over medium heat.
4. Cook the chicken tenders in batches for about 3-4 minutes per side, or until golden brown and cooked through.
5. Transfer to a plate lined with paper towels to drain any excess oil.
6. Serve immediately.

Number of Serves: 4

Nutritional Info per Serving:

- Calories: 350
- Protein: 28g
- Carbohydrates: 10g
- Fiber: 4g
- Sugars: 1g
- Fat: 22g

Cooking Time: 20 minutes

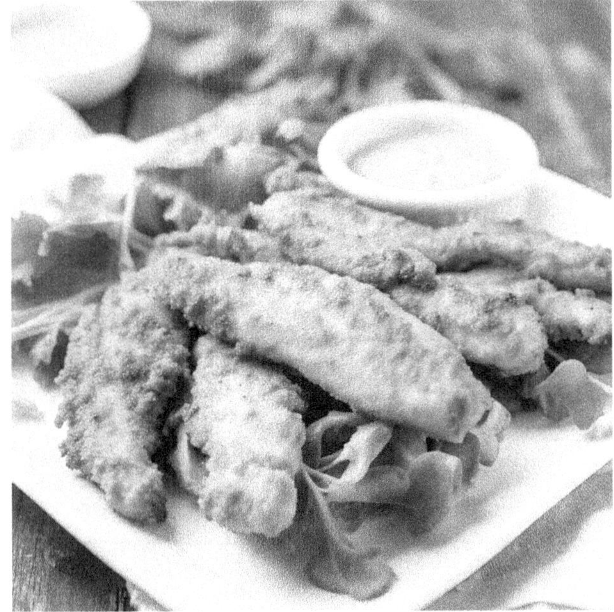

11. Herbed Chicken and Veggie Soup
Ingredients:
- 1 tablespoon olive oil
- 1 onion, chopped
- 2 cloves garlic, minced
- 2 boneless, skinless chicken breasts, diced
- 2 carrots, sliced
- 2 celery stalks, sliced
- 1 zucchini, diced
- 6 cups low-sodium chicken broth
- 1 teaspoon dried thyme
- 1 teaspoon dried rosemary
- 1/4 cup fresh parsley, chopped

Instructions:
1. Heat olive oil in a large pot over medium heat.
2. Add onion and garlic, cooking until softened, about 5 minutes.
3. Add diced chicken breasts and cook until no longer pink, about 5-7 minutes.
4. Add carrots, celery, zucchini, chicken broth, thyme, and rosemary.
5. Bring to a boil, then reduce heat and simmer for 20 minutes, or until the vegetables are tender.
6. Stir in fresh parsley before serving.
7. Serve hot.

Number of Serves: 4
Nutritional Info per Serving:
- Calories: 200
- Protein: 25g
- Carbohydrates: 10g
- Fiber: 3g
- Sugars: 4g
- Fat: 6g

Cooking Time: 35 minutes

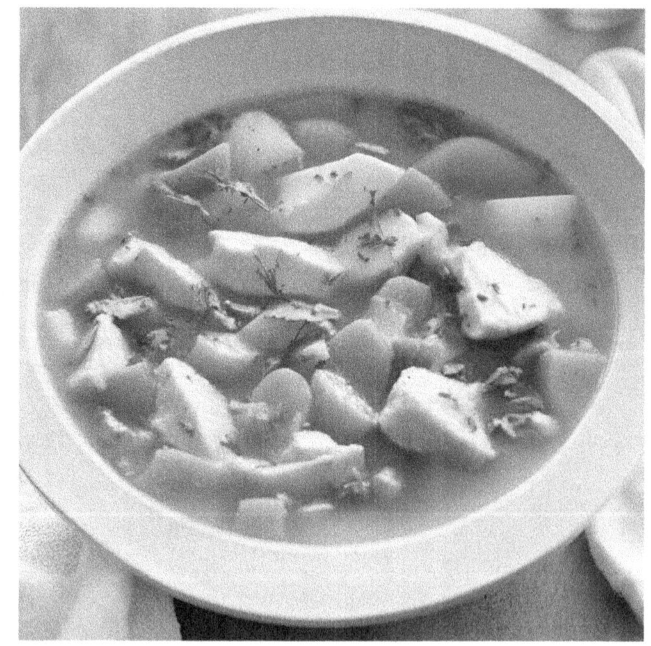

12. Lemon Herb Roasted Chicken

Ingredients:

- 1 whole chicken (about 4 lbs)
- 1/4 cup olive oil
- 1 lemon, sliced
- 4 cloves garlic, minced
- 1 tablespoon fresh thyme, chopped
- 1 tablespoon fresh rosemary, chopped
- 1 tablespoon fresh parsley, chopped

Instructions:

1. Preheat oven to 375°F (190°C).
2. In a small bowl, mix olive oil, minced garlic, thyme, rosemary, and parsley.
3. Rub the herb mixture all over the chicken, including under the skin.
4. Stuff the cavity with lemon slices.
5. Place the chicken in a roasting pan and roast for about 1 hour and 30 minutes, or until the internal temperature reaches 165°F (74°C).
6. Let the chicken rest for 10 minutes before carving.
7. Serve with roasted vegetables or your favorite side dish.

Number of Serves: 6

Nutritional Info per Serving:

- Calories: 320
- Protein: 28g
- Carbohydrates: 2g
- Fiber: 0g
- Sugars: 0g
- Fat: 22g

Cooking Time: 1 hour 45 minutes

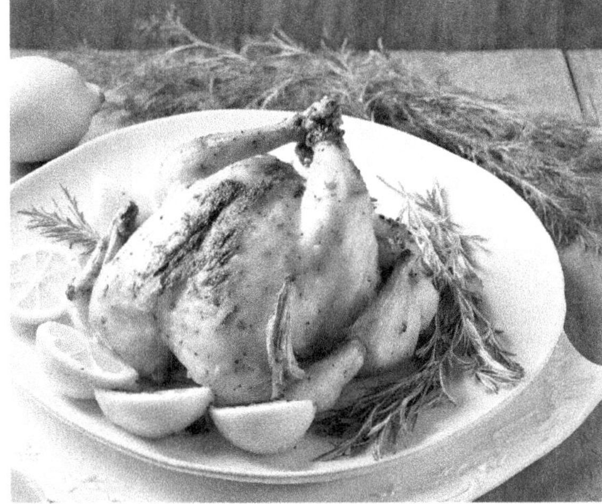

13. Smoky BBQ Chicken

Ingredients:

- 4 boneless, skinless chicken breasts
- 1/2 cup tomato sauce (low-sugar)
- 2 tablespoons apple cider vinegar
- 2 tablespoons honey or maple syrup
- 1 tablespoon smoked paprika
- 1 teaspoon garlic powder
- 1 teaspoon onion powder
- 1/2 teaspoon chili powder

Instructions:

1. Preheat your grill to medium-high heat.
2. In a bowl, mix tomato sauce, apple cider vinegar, honey or maple syrup, smoked paprika, garlic powder, onion powder, and chili powder to make the BBQ sauce.
3. Brush the chicken breasts with the BBQ sauce.
4. Grill the chicken breasts for 6-7 minutes per side, or until fully cooked.
5. Brush with additional BBQ sauce during the last few minutes of grilling.
6. Serve immediately.

Number of Serves: 4

Nutritional Info per Serving:

- Calories: 220
- Protein: 28g
- Carbohydrates: 18g
- Fiber: 1g
- Sugars: 12g
- Fat: 4g

Cooking Time: 20 minutes

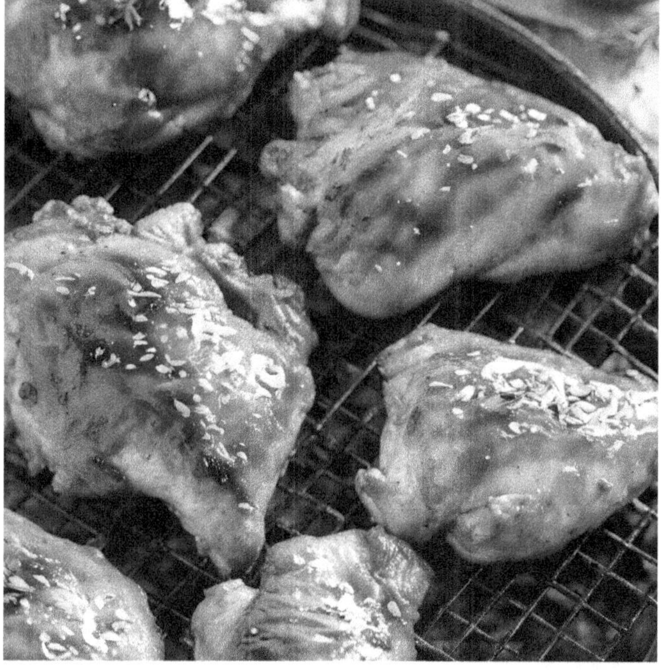

14. Roasted Chicken Drumsticks with Herbs

Ingredients:

- 8 chicken drumsticks
- 2 tablespoons olive oil
- 1 tablespoon fresh rosemary, chopped
- 1 tablespoon fresh thyme, chopped
- 1 tablespoon fresh oregano, chopped
- 3 cloves garlic, minced
- 1 lemon, sliced

Instructions:

1. Preheat oven to 400°F (200°C).
2. In a bowl, mix olive oil, rosemary, thyme, oregano, and minced garlic.
3. Rub the herb mixture all over the chicken drumsticks.
4. Arrange the drumsticks in a single layer on a baking sheet.
5. Place lemon slices around the drumsticks.
6. Roast in the preheated oven for 35-40 minutes, or until the chicken is cooked through and the skin is crispy.
7. Serve immediately.

Number of Serves: 4

Nutritional Info per Serving:

- Calories: 280
- Protein: 28g
- Carbohydrates: 2g
- Fiber: 0g
- Sugars: 0g
- Fat: 18g

Cooking Time: 40 minutes

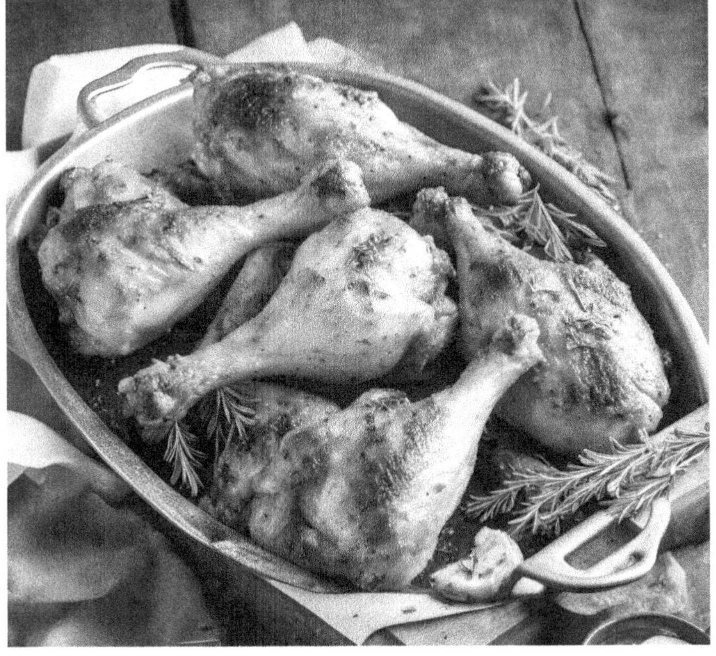

15. Chicken and Spinach Stew
Ingredients:
- 1 tablespoon olive oil
- 1 onion, chopped
- 2 cloves garlic, minced
- 1 lb (450g) boneless, skinless chicken thighs, cut into bite-sized pieces
- 4 cups low-sodium chicken broth
- 1 can (14.5 oz) diced tomatoes
- 2 cups fresh spinach, chopped
- 1 teaspoon dried basil
- 1 teaspoon dried oregano
- 1/2 teaspoon ground turmeric

Instructions:
1. Heat olive oil in a large pot over medium heat.
2. Add onion and garlic, cooking until softened, about 5 minutes.
3. Add chicken thighs and cook until browned, about 5-7 minutes.
4. Stir in chicken broth, diced tomatoes, basil, oregano, and turmeric.
5. Bring to a boil, then reduce heat and simmer for 20 minutes.
6. Stir in chopped spinach and cook for an additional 5 minutes.
7. Serve hot.

Number of Serves: 4
Nutritional Info per Serving:
- Calories: 250
- Protein: 26g
- Carbohydrates: 10g
- Fiber: 3g
- Sugars: 4g
- Fat: 12g

Cooking Time: 35 minutes

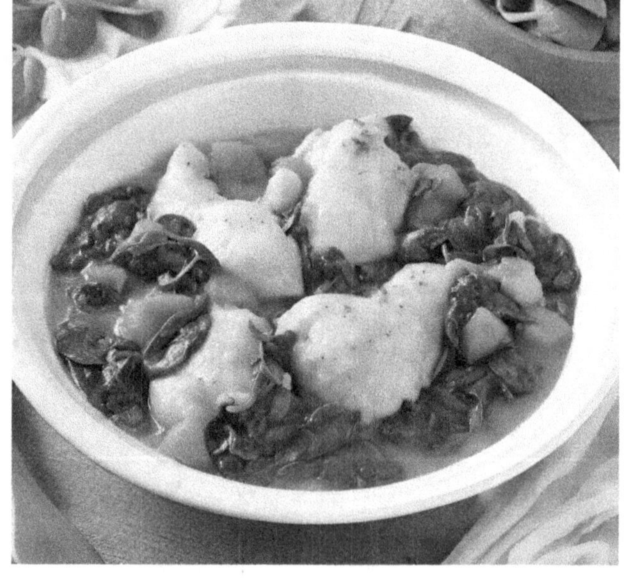

16. Chicken and Mango Salad

Ingredients:

- 2 boneless, skinless chicken breasts
- 1 tablespoon olive oil
- 1 teaspoon ground cumin
- 1 large mango, peeled and diced
- 4 cups mixed salad greens
- 1/4 cup red onion, thinly sliced
- 1/4 cup fresh cilantro, chopped
- 1 avocado, diced
- 2 tablespoons lime juice
- 1 tablespoon honey or maple syrup

Instructions:

1. Preheat grill to medium-high heat.
2. Rub chicken breasts with olive oil and ground cumin.
3. Grill chicken for 6-7 minutes per side, or until fully cooked. Let cool, then slice thinly.
4. In a large bowl, combine mango, salad greens, red onion, cilantro, and avocado.
5. In a small bowl, whisk together lime juice and honey or maple syrup to make the dressing.
6. Add the sliced chicken to the salad and drizzle with dressing.
7. Toss gently to combine and serve immediately.

Number of Serves: 4

Nutritional Info per Serving:

- Calories: 300
- Protein: 26g
- Carbohydrates: 20g
- Fiber: 6g
- Sugars: 12g
- Fat: 14g

Cooking Time: 20 minutes

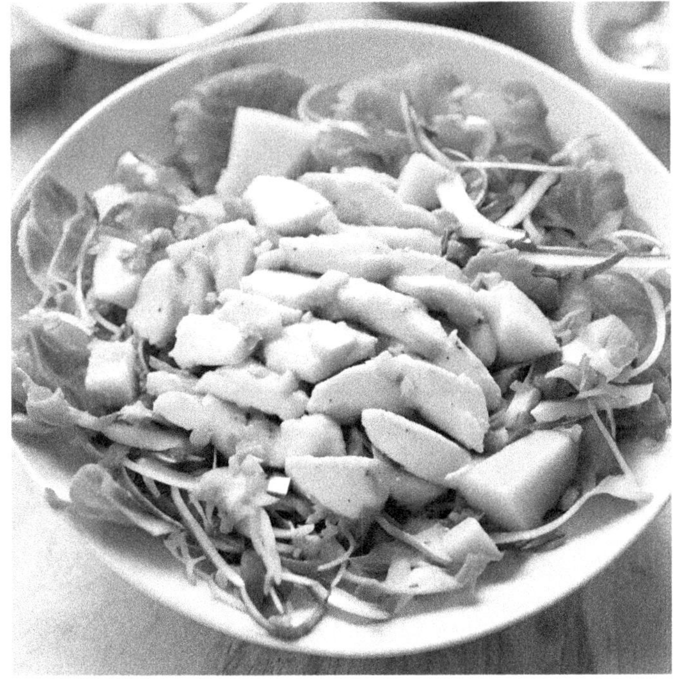

17. Lime and Cilantro Baked Chicken

Ingredients:

- 4 boneless, skinless chicken breasts
- 1/4 cup fresh lime juice
- 2 tablespoons olive oil
- 3 cloves garlic, minced
- 1/4 cup fresh cilantro, chopped
- 1 teaspoon ground cumin

Instructions:

1. Preheat oven to 375°F (190°C).
2. In a small bowl, mix lime juice, olive oil, garlic, cilantro, and cumin.
3. Place chicken breasts in a baking dish and pour the lime mixture over them, ensuring they are well coated.
4. Bake for 25-30 minutes, or until the chicken is cooked through and juices run clear.
5. Serve immediately.

Number of Serves: 4

Nutritional Info per Serving:

- Calories: 220
- Protein: 28g
- Carbohydrates: 3g
- Fiber: 1g
- Sugars: 1g
- Fat: 10g

Cooking Time: 30 minutes

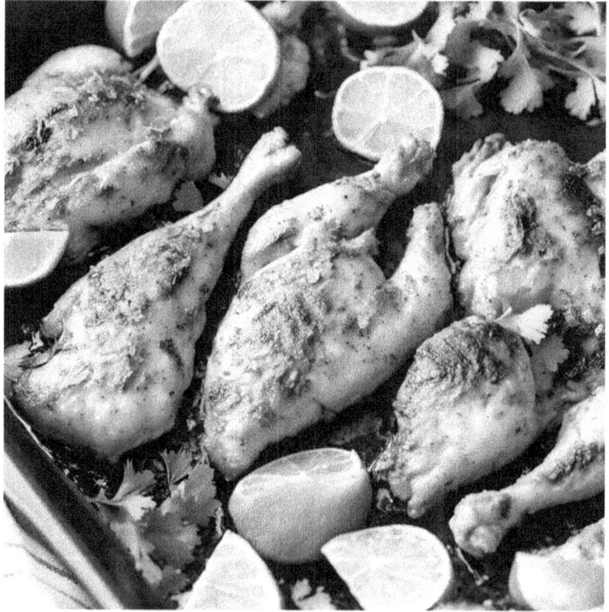

18. Chicken Tikka Masala with Almond Milk

Ingredients:

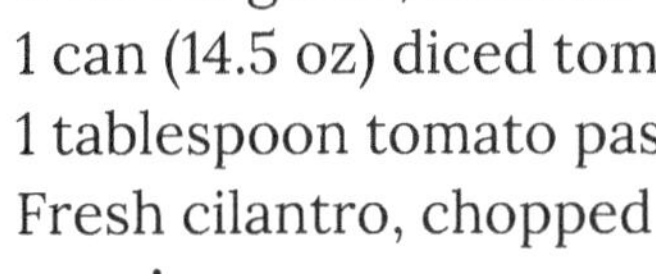

- 1 lb (450g) boneless, skinless chicken breasts, cut into bite-sized pieces
- 1 cup unsweetened almond milk
- 1 cup plain Greek yogurt
- 2 tablespoons lemon juice
- 2 teaspoons ground cumin
- 2 teaspoons ground coriander
- 2 teaspoons ground turmeric
- 1 teaspoon ground paprika
- 1 teaspoon ground garam masala
- 1 teaspoon ground ginger
- 1 tablespoon olive oil
- 1 large onion, chopped
- 3 cloves garlic, minced
- 1 can (14.5 oz) diced tomatoes
- 1 tablespoon tomato paste
- Fresh cilantro, chopped (for garnish)

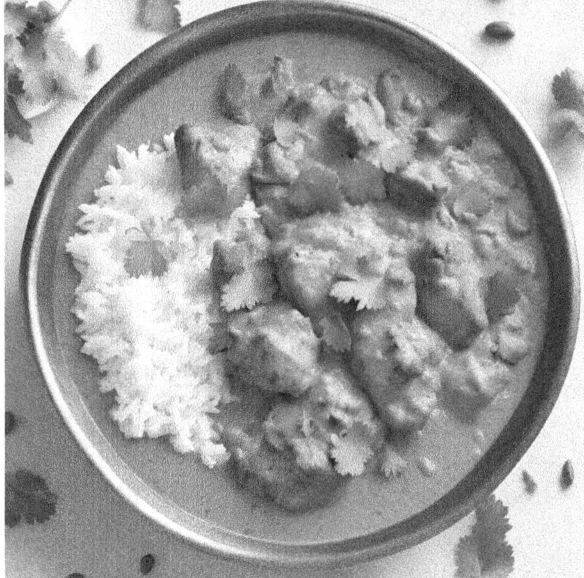

Instructions:

1. In a large bowl, mix Greek yogurt, lemon juice, 1 teaspoon ground cumin, 1 teaspoon ground coriander, and 1 teaspoon turmeric. Add the chicken pieces and coat well. Marinate for at least 1 hour or overnight.
2. Heat olive oil in a large skillet over medium heat. Add onions and cook until softened, about 5 minutes.
3. Add garlic, 1 teaspoon ground cumin, 1 teaspoon ground coriander, turmeric, paprika, garam masala, and ground ginger. Cook for 1-2 minutes until fragrant.
4. Add diced tomatoes, tomato paste, and almond milk. Stir well to combine and bring to a simmer.
5. Add the marinated chicken pieces and cook for 15-20 minutes, or until the chicken is cooked through and the sauce thickens.
6. Garnish with fresh cilantro and serve immediately.

Number of Serves: 4

Nutritional Info per Serving:

- Calories: 300
- Protein: 28g
- Carbohydrates: 14g
- Fiber: 3g
- Sugars: 7g
- Fat: 14g

Cooking Time: 40 minutes (plus marinating time)

19. One-Pan Harissa Chicken

Ingredients:

- 4 boneless, skinless chicken thighs
- 2 tablespoons harissa paste
- 1 tablespoon olive oil
- 1 red onion, sliced
- 1 red bell pepper, sliced
- 1 yellow bell pepper, sliced
- 1 zucchini, sliced
- 1 cup cherry tomatoes
- 1/4 cup fresh parsley, chopped

Instructions:

1. Preheat oven to 400°F (200°C).
2. In a large bowl, toss chicken thighs with harissa paste until well coated.
3. In a large baking dish, combine onion, red and yellow bell peppers, zucchini, and cherry tomatoes. Drizzle with olive oil and toss to coat.
4. Nestle the chicken thighs into the vegetables.
5. Bake for 35-40 minutes, or until the chicken is cooked through and the vegetables are tender.
6. Garnish with fresh parsley and serve immediately.

Number of Serves: 4

Nutritional Info per Serving:

- Calories: 320
- Protein: 25g
- Carbohydrates: 12g
- Fiber: 4g
- Sugars: 6g
- Fat: 20g

Cooking Time: 45 minutes

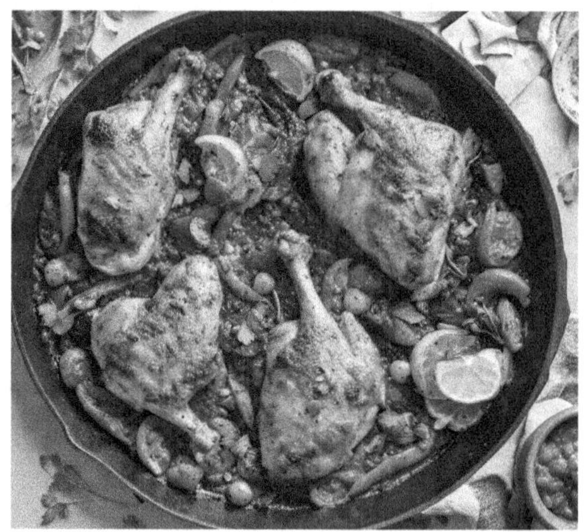

20. Chicken and Broccoli Alfredo with Coconut Cream

Ingredients:

- 1 lb (450g) boneless, skinless chicken breasts, cut into bite-sized pieces
- 2 tablespoons olive oil
- 3 cloves garlic, minced
- 1 head broccoli, cut into florets
- 1 cup unsweetened coconut cream
- 1/4 cup nutritional yeast
- 1 teaspoon dried basil
- 1 teaspoon dried oregano
- 1/2 teaspoon ground nutmeg
- 8 oz (225g) whole grain pasta (optional)
- Fresh parsley, chopped (for garnish)

Instructions:

1. If using pasta, cook according to package instructions. Drain and set aside.
2. In a large skillet, heat olive oil over medium heat. Add chicken pieces and cook until no longer pink, about 5-7 minutes.
3. Add garlic and cook for another 1-2 minutes until fragrant.
4. Add broccoli florets and cook for 5 minutes until tender-crisp.
5. Stir in coconut cream, nutritional yeast, basil, oregano, and nutmeg. Bring to a simmer and cook for 5 minutes until the sauce thickens.
6. If using pasta, add it to the skillet and toss to combine with the sauce.
7. Garnish with fresh parsley and serve immediately.

Number of Serves: 4

Nutritional Info per Serving:

- Calories: 350
- Protein: 28g
- Carbohydrates: 15g
- Fiber: 6g
- Sugars: 3g
- Fat: 22g

Cooking Time: 25 minutes

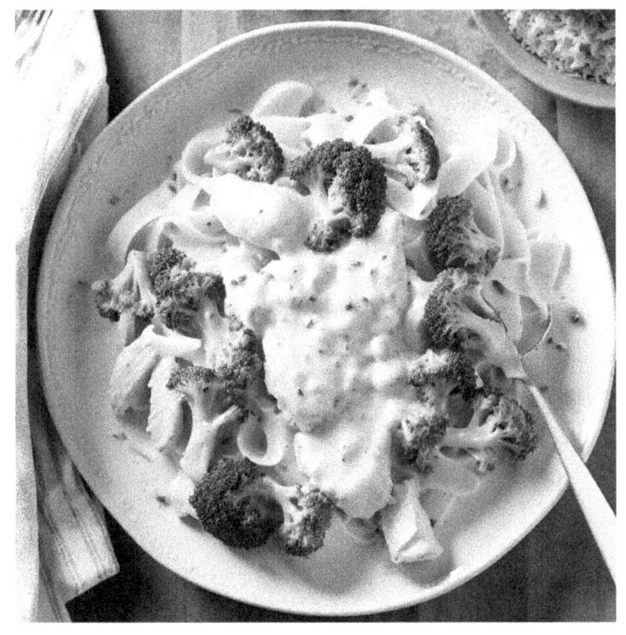

Fish & Seafood Recipes

1. Grilled Salmon with Lemon and Dill
Ingredients:
- 4 salmon fillets (about 6 oz each)
- 2 tablespoons olive oil
- 1 lemon, thinly sliced
- 2 tablespoons fresh dill, chopped
- 3 cloves garlic, minced

Instructions:
1. Preheat the grill to medium-high heat.
2. Brush the salmon fillets with olive oil.
3. Sprinkle minced garlic and fresh dill evenly over the fillets.
4. Place lemon slices on top of each fillet.
5. Grill the salmon for about 4-5 minutes per side, until the salmon is opaque and flakes easily with a fork.
6. Serve immediately.

Number of Serves: 4
Nutritional Info per Serving:
- Calories: 350
- Protein: 34g
- Carbohydrates: 2g
- Fiber: 1g
- Sugars: 0g
- Fat: 22g

Cooking Time: 10 minutes

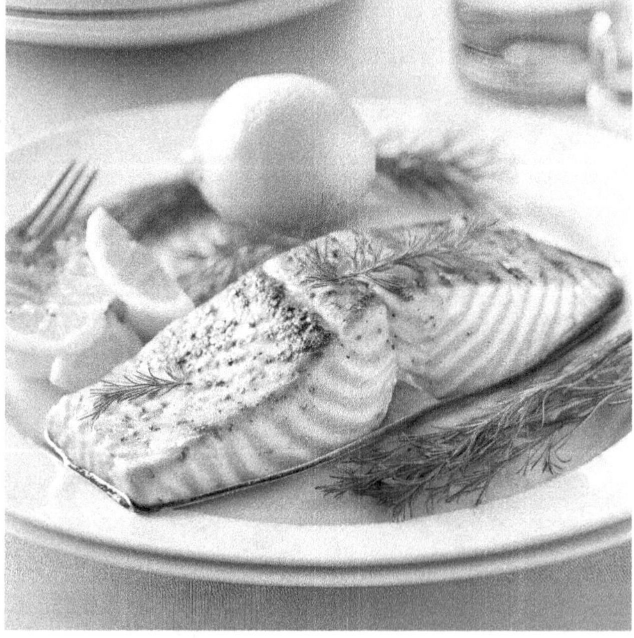

2. Shrimp Stir-Fry with Vegetables

Ingredients:

- 1 lb (450g) shrimp, peeled and deveined
- 2 tablespoons olive oil
- 1 red bell pepper, sliced
- 1 yellow bell pepper, sliced
- 1 cup broccoli florets
- 1 carrot, thinly sliced
- 2 cloves garlic, minced
- 1 tablespoon fresh ginger, grated
- 1/4 cup low-sodium soy sauce or tamari
- 1 tablespoon honey or maple syrup
- 1 tablespoon rice vinegar

Instructions:

1. Heat olive oil in a large skillet or wok over medium-high heat.
2. Add garlic and ginger, and cook for 1-2 minutes until fragrant.
3. Add the shrimp and cook until they turn pink, about 2-3 minutes. Remove and set aside.
4. In the same skillet, add bell peppers, broccoli, and carrot. Stir-fry for about 5-7 minutes until vegetables are tender-crisp.
5. In a small bowl, mix soy sauce or tamari, honey or maple syrup, and rice vinegar.
6. Return the shrimp to the skillet and pour the sauce over. Stir well to combine and cook for another 2-3 minutes.
7. Serve immediately.

Number of Serves: 4

Nutritional Info per Serving:

- Calories: 220
- Protein: 24g
- Carbohydrates: 14g
- Fiber: 3g
- Sugars: 7g
- Fat: 9g

Cooking Time: 15 minutes

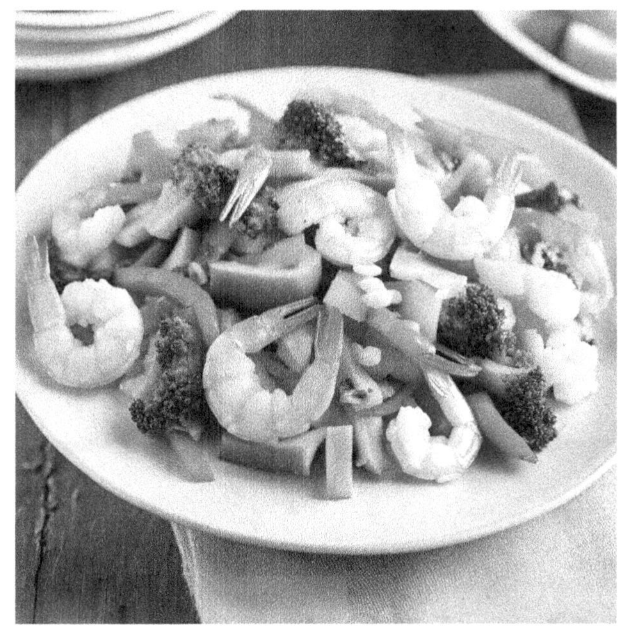

3. Baked Cod with Olive Tapenade

Ingredients:

- 4 cod fillets (about 6 oz each)
- 2 tablespoons olive oil
- 1/2 cup black olives, pitted and chopped
- 2 tablespoons capers, drained
- 1 clove garlic, minced
- 2 tablespoons fresh parsley, chopped
- 1 tablespoon lemon juice

Instructions:

1. Preheat the oven to 375°F (190°C).
2. Place cod fillets in a baking dish and brush with olive oil.
3. In a small bowl, mix black olives, capers, garlic, parsley, and lemon juice to make the tapenade.
4. Spread the olive tapenade evenly over the cod fillets.
5. Bake for 20-25 minutes, or until the cod is cooked through and flakes easily with a fork.
6. Serve immediately.

Number of Serves: 4

Nutritional Info per Serving:

- Calories: 240
- Protein: 30g
- Carbohydrates: 2g
- Fiber: 1g
- Sugars: 0g
- Fat: 12g

Cooking Time: 25 minutes

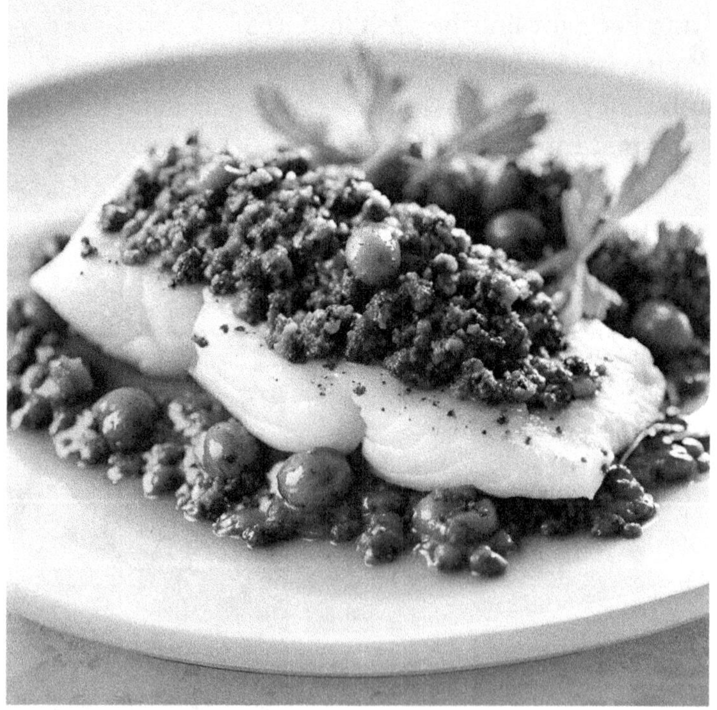

4. Seared Tuna Steak with Avocado Salsa

Ingredients:

- 4 tuna steaks (about 6 oz each)
- 2 tablespoons olive oil
- 1 avocado, diced
- 1 cup cherry tomatoes, halved
- 1/4 cup red onion, finely chopped
- 1/4 cup fresh cilantro, chopped
- 1 tablespoon lime juice

Instructions:

1. Heat olive oil in a large skillet over medium-high heat.
2. Sear the tuna steaks for about 2-3 minutes per side, or until they reach the desired doneness.
3. In a medium bowl, combine avocado, cherry tomatoes, red onion, cilantro, and lime juice to make the salsa.
4. Serve the seared tuna steaks topped with avocado salsa.
5. Serve immediately.

Number of Serves: 4

Nutritional Info per Serving:

- Calories: 320
- Protein: 34g
- Carbohydrates: 6g
- Fiber: 3g
- Sugars: 1g
- Fat: 18g

Cooking Time: 10 minutes

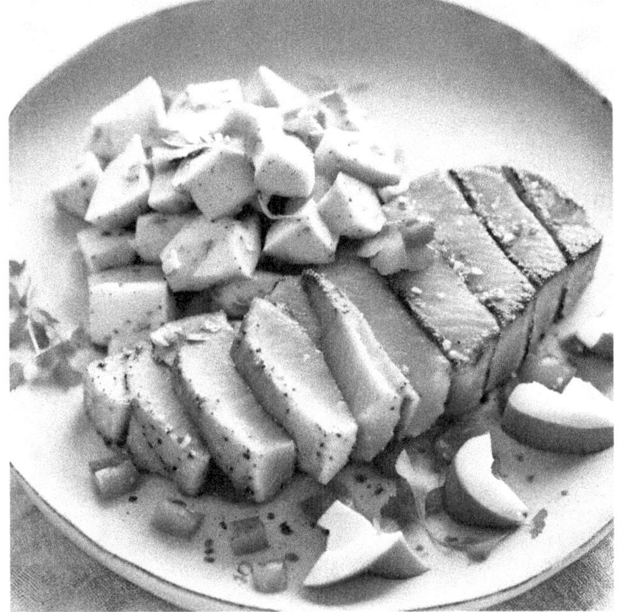

5. Clam Soup with Vegetables

Ingredients:

- 2 tablespoons olive oil
- 1 onion, chopped
- 3 cloves garlic, minced
- 4 cups low-sodium chicken broth
- 1 cup carrots, sliced
- 1 cup celery, sliced
- 2 cups potatoes, diced
- 2 lbs (900g) clams, scrubbed and cleaned
- 1/4 cup fresh parsley, chopped
- 1/2 teaspoon ground turmeric

Instructions:

1. Heat olive oil in a large pot over medium heat.
2. Add onion and garlic, cooking until softened, about 5 minutes.
3. Stir in turmeric and cook for another minute.
4. Add chicken broth, carrots, celery, and potatoes. Bring to a boil.
5. Reduce heat and simmer for about 15 minutes, or until the vegetables are tender.
6. Add the clams and cover the pot. Cook for about 5-7 minutes, or until the clams open. Discard any clams that do not open.
7. Stir in fresh parsley and serve hot.

Number of Serves: 4

Nutritional Info per Serving:

- Calories: 250
- Protein: 24g
- Carbohydrates: 20g
- Fiber: 4g
- Sugars: 5g
- Fat: 10g

Cooking Time: 30 minutes

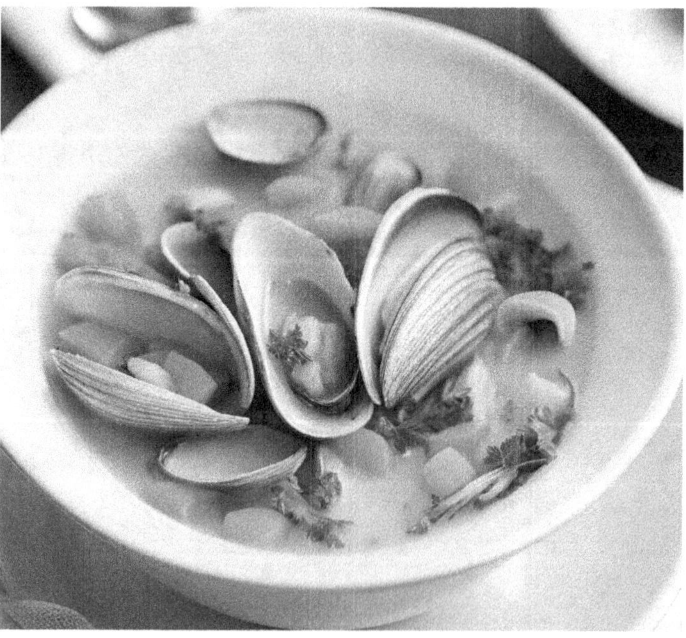

6. Pan-Seared Scallops with Lemon Butter Sauce

Ingredients:

- 1 lb (450g) sea scallops
- 2 tablespoons olive oil
- 3 tablespoons unsalted butter
- 2 cloves garlic, minced
- 1/4 cup fresh lemon juice
- 2 tablespoons fresh parsley, chopped

Instructions:

1. Pat scallops dry with paper towels.
2. Heat olive oil in a large skillet over medium-high heat.
3. Add scallops to the skillet and sear for about 2-3 minutes on each side until golden brown and opaque in the center. Remove scallops and set aside.
4. In the same skillet, add butter and garlic. Cook for about 1 minute until garlic is fragrant.
5. Stir in lemon juice and cook for another 1-2 minutes until the sauce thickens slightly.
6. Return scallops to the skillet and spoon the sauce over them. Cook for an additional minute to heat through.
7. Sprinkle with fresh parsley and serve immediately.

Number of Serves: 4

Nutritional Info per Serving:

- Calories: 250
- Protein: 20g
- Carbohydrates: 3g
- Fiber: 0g
- Sugars: 0g
- Fat: 18g

Cooking Time: 15 minutes

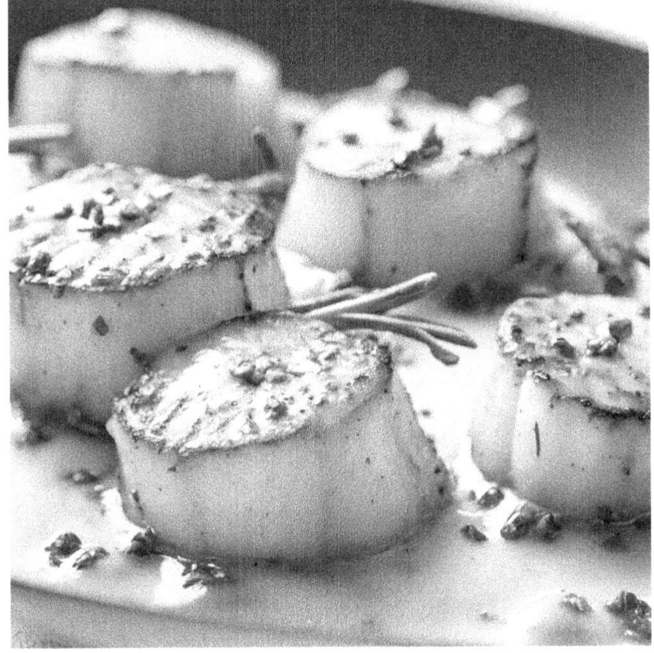

7. Salmon and Quinoa Salad

Ingredients:

- 1 lb (450g) salmon fillet
- 1 cup quinoa, rinsed
- 2 cups water
- 2 tablespoons olive oil
- 1 lemon, juiced
- 1 cup cherry tomatoes, halved
- 1 cucumber, diced
- 1/4 cup red onion, finely chopped
- 1/4 cup fresh parsley, chopped

Instructions:

1. Preheat oven to 375°F (190°C).
2. Place salmon on a baking sheet and bake for 15-20 minutes until cooked through. Let cool and flake with a fork.
3. In a saucepan, bring quinoa and water to a boil. Reduce heat, cover, and simmer for 15 minutes until water is absorbed and quinoa is tender. Let cool.
4. In a large bowl, combine cooked quinoa, flaked salmon, cherry tomatoes, cucumber, red onion, and parsley.
5. In a small bowl, whisk together olive oil and lemon juice.
6. Pour the dressing over the salad and toss to combine.
7. Serve immediately or chill in the refrigerator until ready to serve.

Number of Serves: 4

Nutritional Info per Serving:

- Calories: 350
- Protein: 28g
- Carbohydrates: 30g
- Fiber: 5g
- Sugars: 3g
- Fat: 14g

Cooking Time: 35 minutes

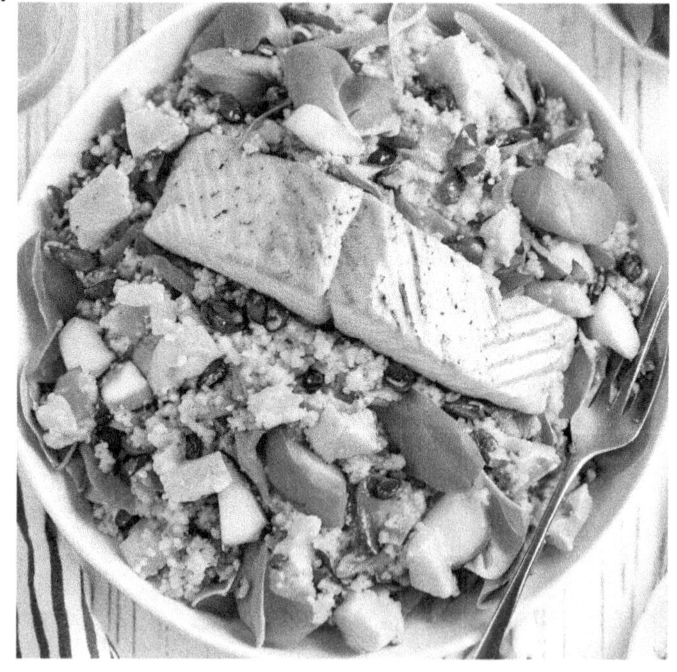

8. Prawn Cocktail with Avocado

Ingredients:

- 1 lb (450g) cooked prawns, peeled and deveined
- 2 avocados, diced
- 1/4 cup red onion, finely chopped
- 1/4 cup fresh cilantro, chopped
- 1 tablespoon lime juice
- 1/2 cup cocktail sauce

Instructions:

1. In a large bowl, combine cooked prawns, diced avocados, red onion, cilantro, and lime juice.
2. Gently toss to mix.
3. Divide the prawn mixture into serving glasses or bowls.
4. Top each serving with cocktail sauce.
5. Serve immediately.

Number of Serves: 4

Nutritional Info per Serving:

- Calories: 250
- Protein: 22g
- Carbohydrates: 12g
- Fiber: 6g
- Sugars: 6g
- Fat: 14g

Cooking Time: 10 minutes

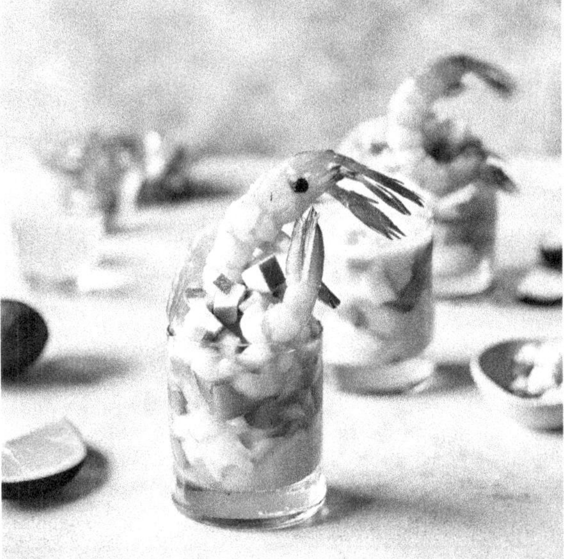

9. Herb-Crusted Halibut

Ingredients:

- 4 halibut fillets (about 6 oz each)
- 1/2 cup almond flour
- 1/4 cup fresh parsley, chopped
- 1/4 cup fresh basil, chopped
- 2 tablespoons fresh thyme, chopped
- 2 tablespoons olive oil
- 2 cloves garlic, minced
- 1 lemon, cut into wedges

Instructions:

1. Preheat oven to 400°F (200°C).
2. In a bowl, combine almond flour, parsley, basil, thyme, and garlic.
3. Brush each halibut fillet with olive oil.
4. Press the herb mixture onto the top of each fillet.
5. Place the fillets on a baking sheet and bake for 15-20 minutes, or until the fish is opaque and flakes easily with a fork.
6. Serve with lemon wedges.

Number of Serves: 4

Nutritional Info per Serving:

- Calories: 320
- Protein: 34g
- Carbohydrates: 4g
- Fiber: 2g
- Sugars: 0g
- Fat: 18g

Cooking Time: 20 minutes

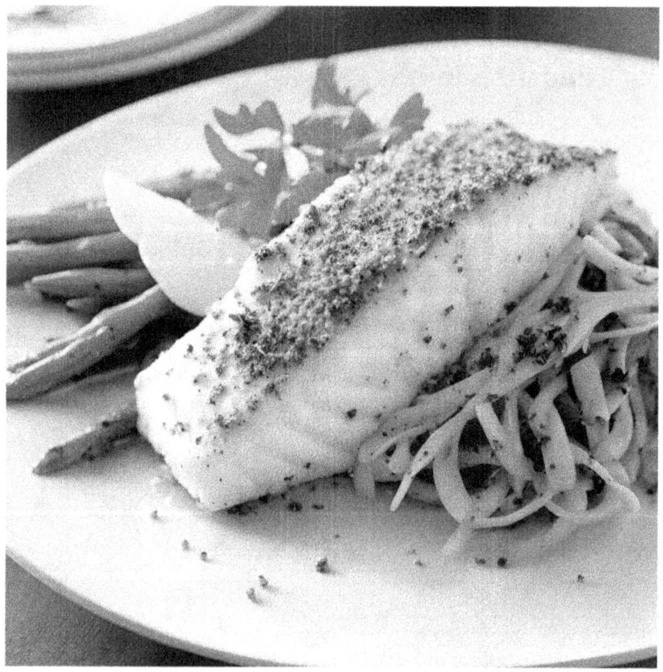

10. Oysters with Mignonette Sauce

Ingredients:

- 12 fresh oysters, shucked
- 1/4 cup red wine vinegar
- 2 tablespoons shallots, finely chopped
- 1 tablespoon fresh lemon juice
- 1 tablespoon fresh parsley, chopped

Instructions:

1. Arrange the shucked oysters on a platter.
2. In a small bowl, combine red wine vinegar, shallots, lemon juice, and parsley to make the mignonette sauce.
3. Spoon a small amount of mignonette sauce onto each oyster.
4. Serve immediately.

Number of Serves: 4

Nutritional Info per Serving:

- Calories: 60
- Protein: 5g
- Carbohydrates: 2g
- Fiber: 0g
- Sugars: 0g
- Fat: 2g

Cooking Time: 10 minutes

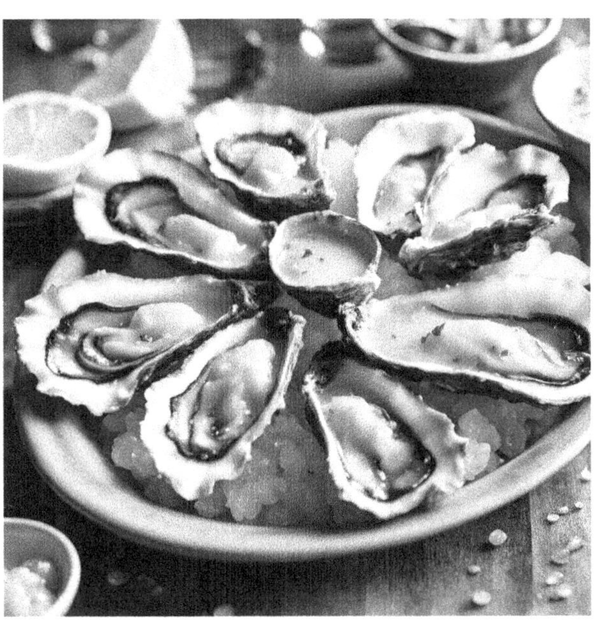

11. Tilapia with Mango Salsa
Ingredients:
- 4 tilapia fillets (about 6 oz each)
- 2 tablespoons olive oil
- 1 mango, peeled and diced
- 1/2 red bell pepper, diced
- 1/4 cup red onion, finely chopped
- 1/4 cup fresh cilantro, chopped
- 1 tablespoon lime juice

Instructions:
1. Preheat oven to 375°F (190°C).
2. Brush the tilapia fillets with olive oil and place them on a baking sheet.
3. Bake for 15-20 minutes, or until the fish is opaque and flakes easily with a fork.
4. While the fish is baking, prepare the mango salsa by combining mango, red bell pepper, red onion, cilantro, and lime juice in a bowl.
5. Serve the baked tilapia topped with mango salsa.

Number of Serves: 4
Nutritional Info per Serving:
- Calories: 220
- Protein: 28g
- Carbohydrates: 12g
- Fiber: 2g
- Sugars: 8g
- Fat: 8g

Cooking Time: 20 minutes

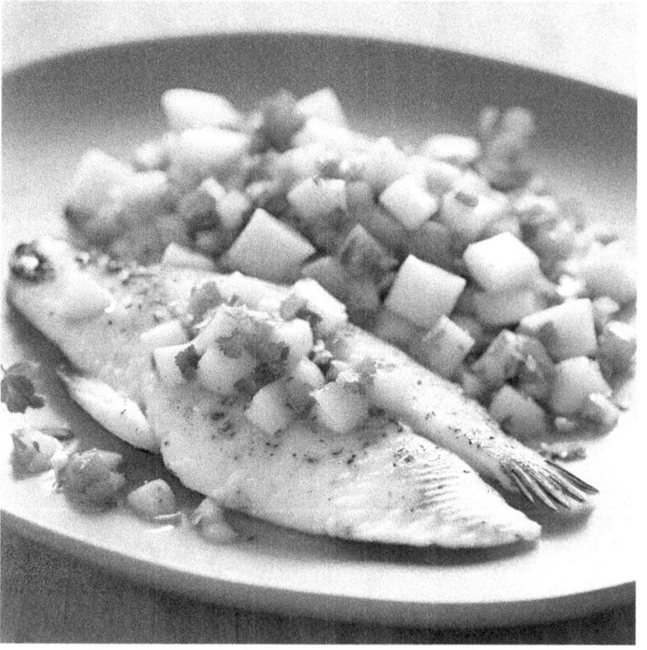

12. Ceviche with Citrus and Cilantro

Ingredients:

- 1 lb (450g) fresh white fish (such as sea bass or tilapia), diced
- 1/2 cup fresh lime juice
- 1/2 cup fresh lemon juice
- 1/4 cup fresh orange juice
- 1 small red onion, finely chopped
- 1 jalapeño, seeded and finely chopped
- 1/4 cup fresh cilantro, chopped
- 1 avocado, diced
- 1 cucumber, diced

Instructions:

1. In a large bowl, combine the diced fish and citrus juices. Cover and refrigerate for at least 1 hour, or until the fish is opaque and "cooked" through.
2. Add the red onion, jalapeño, cilantro, avocado, and cucumber to the fish mixture. Stir gently to combine.
3. Serve immediately, garnished with additional cilantro if desired.

Number of Serves: 4

Nutritional Info per Serving:

- Calories: 180
- Protein: 22g
- Carbohydrates: 10g
- Fiber: 4g
- Sugars: 3g
- Fat: 7g

Cooking Time: 1 hour (including marinating time)

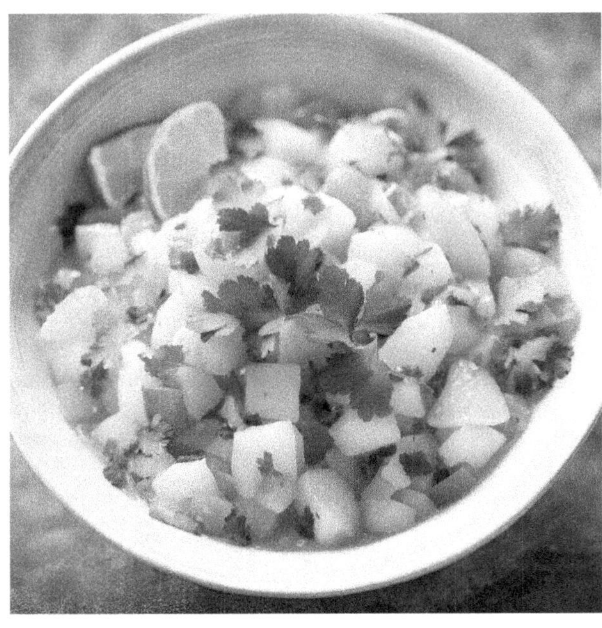

13. Lobster Salad with Mixed Greens

Ingredients:

- 2 lobster tails, cooked and chopped
- 4 cups mixed salad greens
- 1 avocado, sliced
- 1 cup cherry tomatoes, halved
- 1/4 cup red onion, thinly sliced
- 2 tablespoons fresh lemon juice
- 2 tablespoons olive oil
- 1 tablespoon fresh dill, chopped

Instructions:

1. In a large bowl, combine mixed salad greens, avocado, cherry tomatoes, and red onion.
2. Add the chopped lobster to the salad.
3. In a small bowl, whisk together lemon juice, olive oil, and dill.
4. Pour the dressing over the salad and toss gently to combine.
5. Serve immediately.

Number of Serves: 2

Nutritional Info per Serving:

- Calories: 300
- Protein: 20g
- Carbohydrates: 12g
- Fiber: 6g
- Sugars: 4g
- Fat: 20g

Cooking Time: 15 minutes

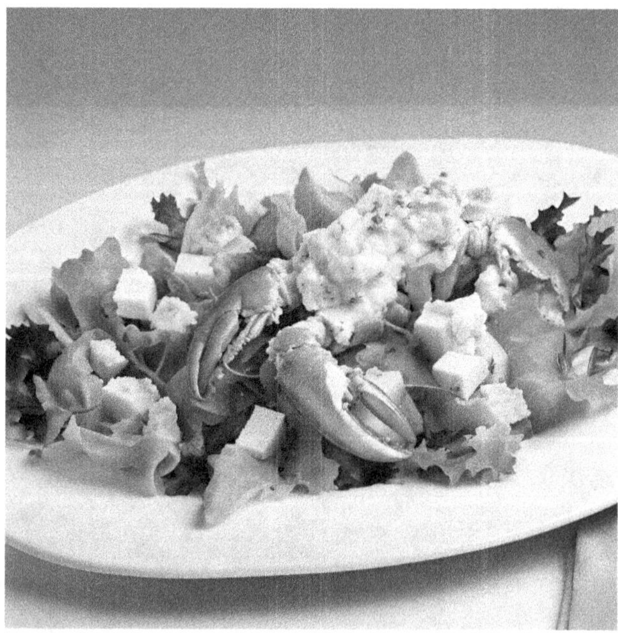

14. Baked Trout with Almonds

Ingredients:
- 4 trout fillets (about 6 oz each)
- 1/4 cup sliced almonds
- 2 tablespoons olive oil
- 1 tablespoon lemon juice
- 1 tablespoon fresh parsley, chopped

Instructions:
1. Preheat oven to 375°F (190°C).
2. Place the trout fillets in a baking dish and drizzle with olive oil and lemon juice.
3. Sprinkle sliced almonds over the top of the fillets.
4. Bake for 15-20 minutes, or until the trout is cooked through and flakes easily with a fork.
5. Garnish with fresh parsley and serve immediately.

Number of Serves: 4

Nutritional Info per Serving:
- Calories: 250
- Protein: 30g
- Carbohydrates: 2g
- Fiber: 1g
- Sugars: 0g
- Fat: 14g

Cooking Time: 20 minutes

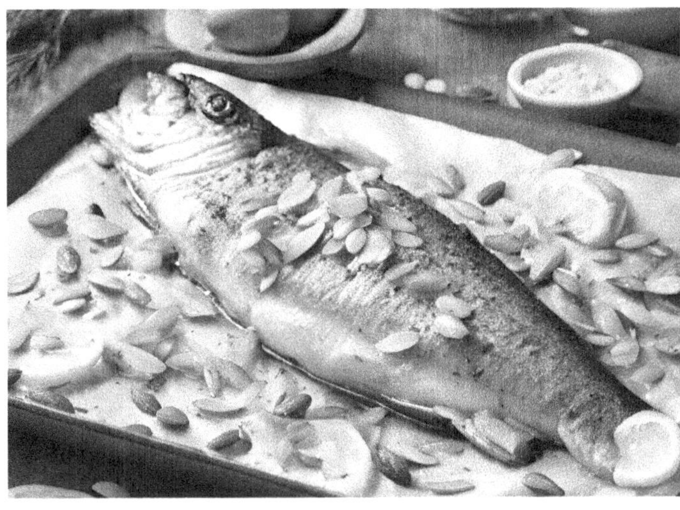

15. Smoked Salmon and Cucumber Rolls

Ingredients:

- 8 oz (225g) smoked salmon, thinly sliced
- 1 large cucumber, thinly sliced lengthwise
- 1 avocado, thinly sliced
- 2 tablespoons fresh dill, chopped
- 1 tablespoon lemon juice

Instructions:

1. Lay the cucumber slices flat on a cutting board.
2. Place a slice of smoked salmon on each cucumber slice.
3. Add a slice of avocado on top of the salmon.
4. Sprinkle with fresh dill and a drizzle of lemon juice.
5. Roll up the cucumber slices and secure with a toothpick if needed.
6. Serve immediately.

Number of Serves: 4

Nutritional Info per Serving:

- Calories: 150
- Protein: 10g
- Carbohydrates: 5g
- Fiber: 3g
- Sugars: 1g
- Fat: 10g

Cooking Time: 10 minutes

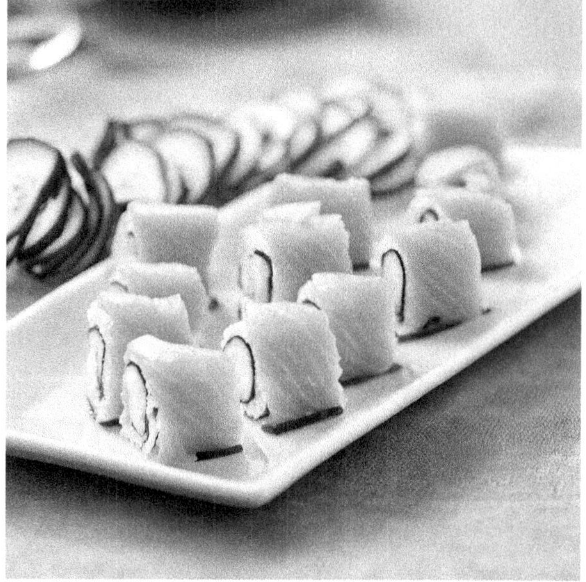

16. Paella with Seafood

Ingredients:

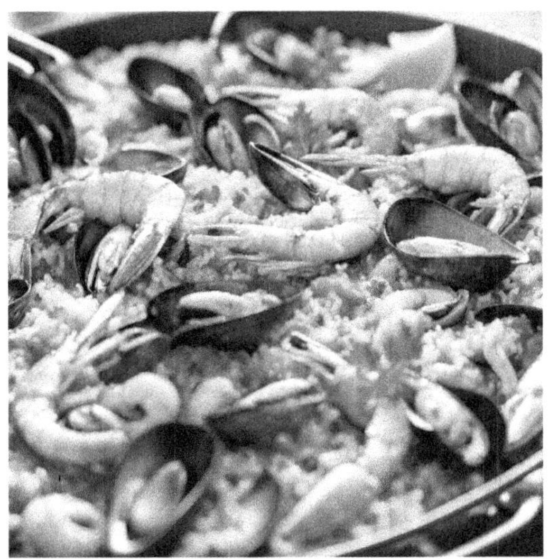

- 1 tablespoon olive oil
- 1 onion, chopped
- 3 cloves garlic, minced
- 1 red bell pepper, chopped
- 1 cup Arborio rice
- 1/2 teaspoon ground turmeric
- 1/2 teaspoon smoked paprika
- 1 can (14.5 oz) diced tomatoes
- 2 cups low-sodium chicken broth
- 1/2 lb (225g) shrimp, peeled and deveined
- 1/2 lb (225g) mussels, cleaned
- 1/2 lb (225g) clams, cleaned
- 1/2 cup frozen peas
- 1/4 cup fresh parsley, chopped

Instructions:

1. Heat olive oil in a large skillet or paella pan over medium heat.
2. Add onion, garlic, and red bell pepper. Cook until softened, about 5 minutes.
3. Stir in Arborio rice, turmeric, and smoked paprika. Cook for 1-2 minutes until the rice is well coated.
4. Add diced tomatoes and chicken broth. Bring to a simmer and cook for about 15 minutes, stirring occasionally.
5. Add shrimp, mussels, and clams. Cover and cook for another 10 minutes, or until the seafood is cooked through and the mussels and clams have opened.
6. Stir in frozen peas and cook for an additional 2 minutes.
7. Garnish with fresh parsley and serve immediately.

Number of Serves: 4

Nutritional Info per Serving:

- Calories: 350
- Protein: 28g
- Carbohydrates: 45g
- Fiber: 5g
- Sugars: 6g
- Fat: 8g

Cooking Time: 35 minutes

17. Grilled Octopus with Olive Oil and Lemon

Ingredients:

- 2 lbs (900g) octopus, cleaned
- 1/4 cup olive oil
- 1/4 cup fresh lemon juice
- 2 cloves garlic, minced
- 1 tablespoon fresh oregano, chopped

Instructions:

1. Bring a large pot of water to a boil. Add the octopus and cook for about 45 minutes until tender. Drain and let cool.
2. Preheat the grill to medium-high heat.
3. Cut the octopus into large pieces.
4. In a bowl, mix olive oil, lemon juice, garlic, and oregano.
5. Brush the octopus pieces with the olive oil mixture.
6. Grill the octopus for about 4-5 minutes per side until charred and heated through.
7. Serve immediately.

Number of Serves: 4

Nutritional Info per Serving:

- Calories: 220
- Protein: 28g
- Carbohydrates: 3g
- Fiber: 1g
- Sugars: 0g
- Fat: 10g

Cooking Time: 55 minutes (including boiling time)

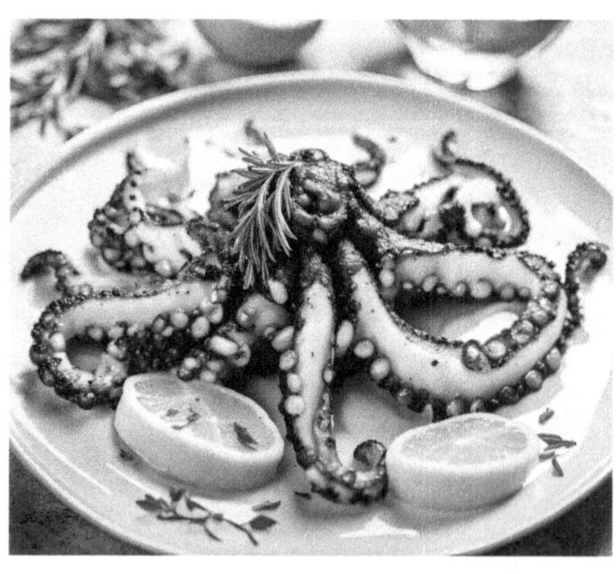

18. Scallop Carpaccio with Citrus Vinaigrette

Ingredients:

- 1 lb (450g) sea scallops, thinly sliced
- 1/4 cup fresh lemon juice
- 1/4 cup fresh orange juice
- 2 tablespoons olive oil
- 1 tablespoon fresh dill, chopped
- 1 tablespoon fresh chives, chopped

Instructions:

1. Arrange the thinly sliced scallops on a serving platter.
2. In a small bowl, whisk together lemon juice, orange juice, and olive oil.
3. Drizzle the citrus vinaigrette over the scallops.
4. Sprinkle with fresh dill and chives.
5. Serve immediately.

Number of Serves: 4

Nutritional Info per Serving:

- Calories: 180
- Protein: 22g
- Carbohydrates: 4g
- Fiber: 0g
- Sugars: 2g
- Fat: 8g

Cooking Time: 10 minutes

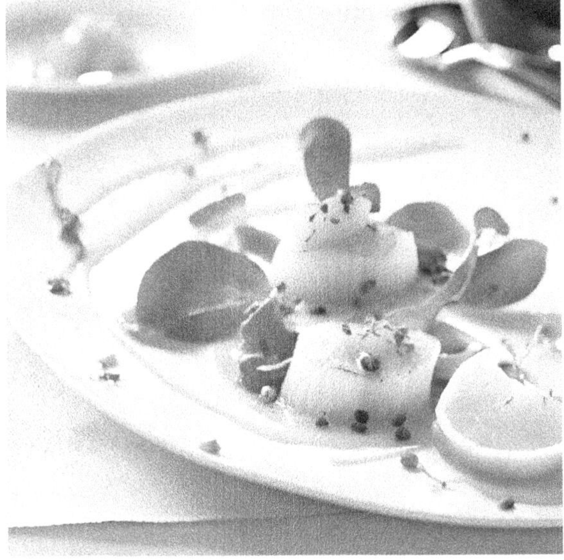

19. Steamed Fish with Ginger and Scallions
Ingredients:
- 4 white fish fillets (such as tilapia or sea bass)
- 2 tablespoons fresh ginger, julienned
- 4 scallions, cut into 2-inch pieces
- 2 tablespoons soy sauce or tamari
- 1 tablespoon rice vinegar
- 1 tablespoon sesame oil

Instructions:
1. Place the fish fillets on a heatproof plate that fits into your steamer.
2. Sprinkle the ginger and scallions over the fish.
3. In a small bowl, mix the soy sauce or tamari, rice vinegar, and sesame oil.
4. Drizzle the mixture over the fish.
5. Steam the fish over boiling water for about 10-12 minutes, or until the fish is opaque and flakes easily with a fork.
6. Serve immediately.

Number of Serves: 4
Nutritional Info per Serving:
- Calories: 180
- Protein: 28g
- Carbohydrates: 2g
- Fiber: 0g
- Sugars: 0g
- Fat: 7g

Cooking Time: 15 minutes

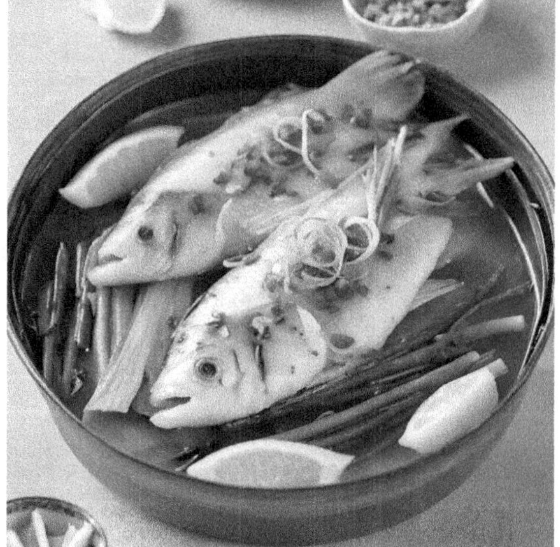

20. Cajun-style Catfish

Ingredients:

- 4 catfish fillets
- 2 tablespoons olive oil
- 1 teaspoon paprika
- 1 teaspoon garlic powder
- 1 teaspoon onion powder
- 1/2 teaspoon dried thyme
- 1/2 teaspoon dried oregano
- 1/4 teaspoon cayenne pepper

Instructions:

1. Preheat the oven to 375°F (190°C).
2. In a small bowl, mix paprika, garlic powder, onion powder, thyme, oregano, and cayenne pepper.
3. Brush the catfish fillets with olive oil.
4. Rub the spice mixture evenly over both sides of the fillets.
5. Place the fillets on a baking sheet and bake for 15-20 minutes, or until the fish is opaque and flakes easily with a fork.
6. Serve immediately.

Number of Serves: 4

Nutritional Info per Serving:

- Calories: 220
- Protein: 24g
- Carbohydrates: 2g
- Fiber: 0g
- Sugars: 0g
- Fat: 12g

Cooking Time: 20 minutes

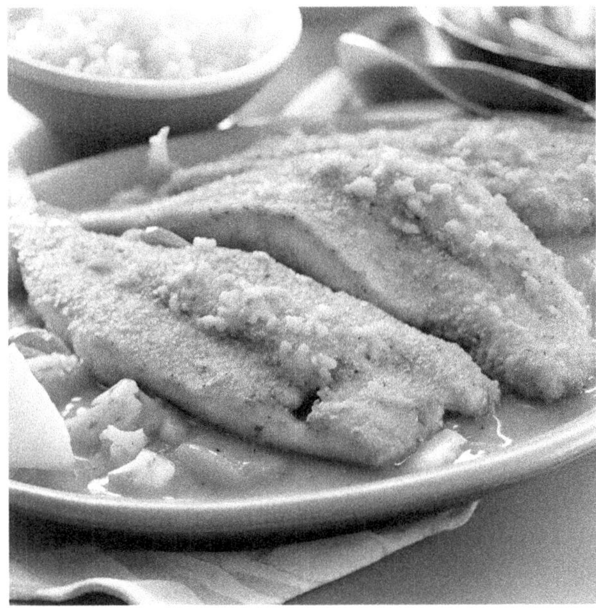

21. Sardines Grilled with Herbs

Ingredients:

- 8 fresh sardines, cleaned
- 2 tablespoons olive oil
- 2 tablespoons fresh parsley, chopped
- 2 tablespoons fresh thyme, chopped
- 1 clove garlic, minced
- 1 lemon, sliced

Instructions:

1. Preheat the grill to medium-high heat.
2. In a small bowl, mix olive oil, parsley, thyme, and garlic.
3. Brush the sardines with the herb mixture.
4. Place the sardines on the grill and cook for about 3-4 minutes per side, until the skin is crispy and the fish is cooked through.
5. Serve with lemon slices.

Number of Serves: 4

Nutritional Info per Serving:

- Calories: 180
- Protein: 24g
- Carbohydrates: 0g
- Fiber: 0g
- Sugars: 0g
- Fat: 9g

Cooking Time: 10 minutes

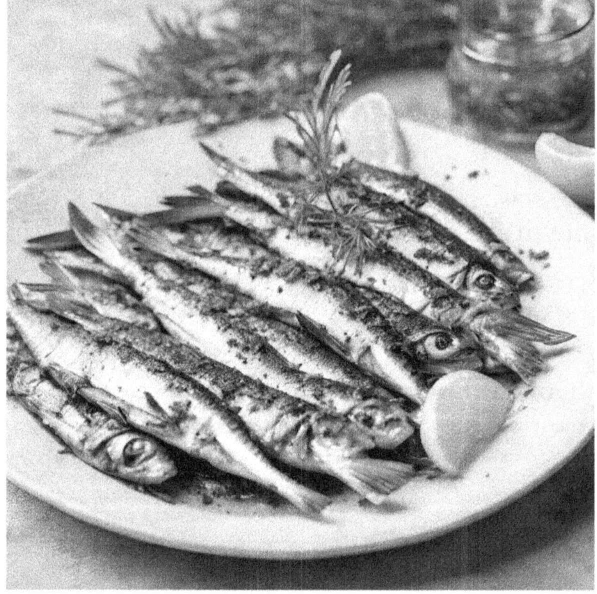

22. Grilled Mahi-Mahi with Pineapple Salsa

Ingredients:

- 4 mahi-mahi fillets
- 2 tablespoons olive oil
- 1 cup fresh pineapple, diced
- 1/4 cup red onion, finely chopped
- 1 jalapeño, seeded and finely chopped
- 1/4 cup fresh cilantro, chopped
- 2 tablespoons lime juice

Instructions:

1. Preheat the grill to medium-high heat.
2. Brush the mahi-mahi fillets with olive oil.
3. Grill the fillets for about 4-5 minutes per side, or until the fish is opaque and flakes easily with a fork.
4. In a medium bowl, combine pineapple, red onion, jalapeño, cilantro, and lime juice to make the salsa.
5. Serve the grilled mahi-mahi topped with pineapple salsa.

Number of Serves: 4

Nutritional Info per Serving:

- Calories: 240
- Protein: 30g
- Carbohydrates: 10g
- Fiber: 2g
- Sugars: 6g
- Fat: 10g

Cooking Time: 15 minutes

23. Pesto Shrimp Pasta

Ingredients:

- 1 lb (450g) shrimp, peeled and deveined
- 8 oz (225g) whole grain pasta
- 1/2 cup pesto sauce (store-bought or homemade)
- 1 tablespoon olive oil
- 1 cup cherry tomatoes, halved
- 1/4 cup pine nuts, toasted (optional)

Instructions:

1. Cook the pasta according to package instructions. Drain and set aside.
2. Heat olive oil in a large skillet over medium heat.
3. Add the shrimp and cook until pink and opaque, about 2-3 minutes per side.
4. Add the cherry tomatoes and cook for an additional 2 minutes.
5. Remove from heat and stir in the cooked pasta and pesto sauce until well combined.
6. Serve immediately, topped with toasted pine nuts if desired.

Number of Serves: 4

Nutritional Info per Serving:

- Calories: 450
- Protein: 28g
- Carbohydrates: 50g
- Fiber: 6g
- Sugars: 4g
- Fat: 16g

Cooking Time: 20 minutes

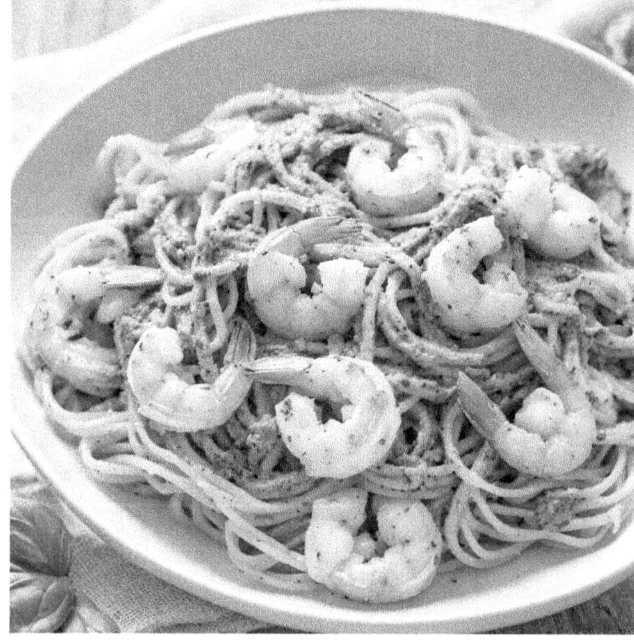

24. Salmon Foil Packets with Vegetables

Ingredients:

- 4 salmon fillets (about 6 oz each)
- 2 zucchinis, sliced
- 1 red bell pepper, sliced
- 1 yellow bell pepper, sliced
- 1 red onion, sliced
- 4 cloves garlic, minced
- 4 tablespoons olive oil
- 4 tablespoons fresh lemon juice
- 2 tablespoons fresh dill, chopped

Instructions:

1. Preheat oven to 375°F (190°C).
2. Prepare 4 large pieces of aluminum foil.
3. Place a salmon fillet in the center of each piece of foil.
4. Divide the zucchini, bell peppers, and onion evenly among the foil packets.
5. Sprinkle minced garlic over the vegetables and salmon.
6. Drizzle each packet with 1 tablespoon of olive oil and 1 tablespoon of lemon juice.
7. Sprinkle fresh dill over each packet.
8. Fold the foil over the salmon and vegetables to create a sealed packet.
9. Bake for 20-25 minutes, or until the salmon is cooked through and the vegetables are tender.
10. Serve immediately.

Number of Serves: 4

Nutritional Info per Serving:

- Calories: 350
- Protein: 28g
- Carbohydrates: 12g
- Fiber: 4g
- Sugars: 6g
- Fat: 22g

Cooking Time: 25 minutes

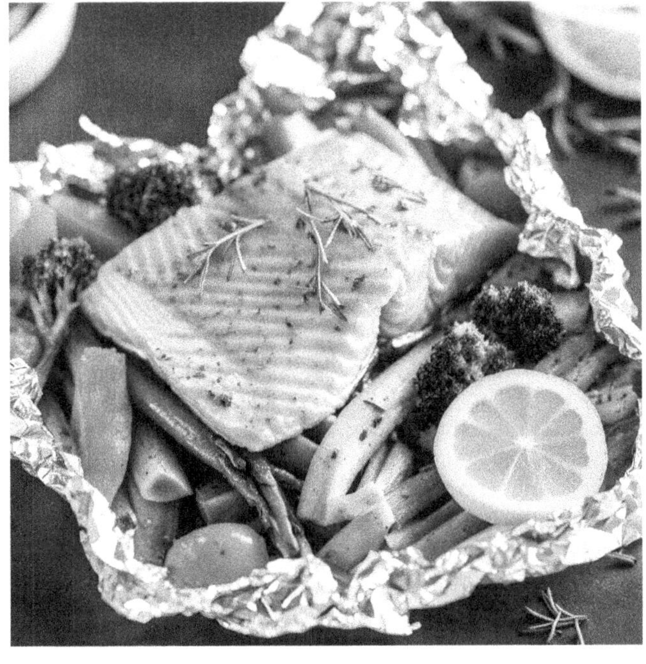

25. Baked Lemon Sole

Ingredients:

- 4 sole fillets (about 6 oz each)
- 3 tablespoons olive oil
- 2 tablespoons fresh lemon juice
- 1 teaspoon dried oregano
- 2 cloves garlic, minced
- 1 lemon, sliced

Instructions:

1. Preheat oven to 375°F (190°C).
2. Place the sole fillets in a baking dish.
3. In a small bowl, mix olive oil, lemon juice, oregano, and minced garlic.
4. Pour the mixture over the sole fillets.
5. Arrange lemon slices on top of the fillets.
6. Bake for 15-20 minutes, or until the fish is opaque and flakes easily with a fork.
7. Serve immediately.

Number of Serves: 4

Nutritional Info per Serving:

- Calories: 200
- Protein: 30g
- Carbohydrates: 3g
- Fiber: 1g
- Sugars: 1g
- Fat: 8g

Cooking Time: 20 minutes

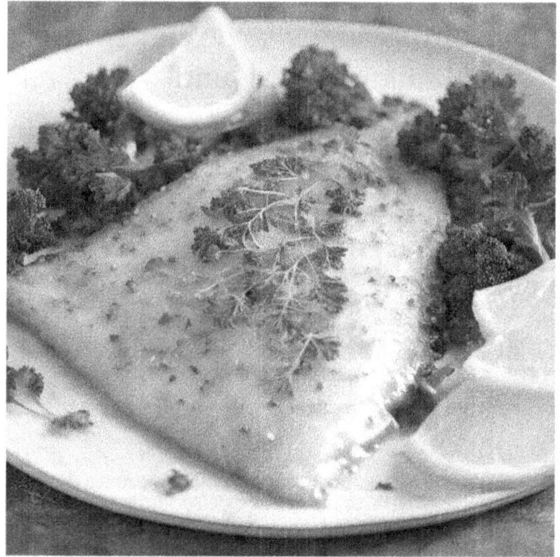

26. Spicy Seafood Soup

Ingredients:

- 1 tablespoon olive oil
- 1 onion, chopped
- 3 cloves garlic, minced
- 1 red bell pepper, chopped
- 1 jalapeño, seeded and chopped
- 1 can (14.5 oz) diced tomatoes
- 4 cups low-sodium fish or vegetable broth
- 1 teaspoon smoked paprika
- 1/2 teaspoon cayenne pepper (optional)
- 1 lb (450g) shrimp, peeled and deveined
- 1/2 lb (225g) white fish fillets (such as cod or halibut), cut into chunks
- 1/2 lb (225g) mussels, cleaned
- 1/2 lb (225g) clams, cleaned
- 1/4 cup fresh cilantro, chopped
- 2 tablespoons fresh lime juice

Instructions:

1. Heat olive oil in a large pot over medium heat.
2. Add onion, garlic, red bell pepper, and jalapeño. Cook until softened, about 5 minutes.
3. Stir in diced tomatoes, broth, smoked paprika, and cayenne pepper if using. Bring to a simmer.
4. Add shrimp, white fish, mussels, and clams to the pot. Cover and cook for about 5-7 minutes, or until the mussels and clams have opened and the seafood is cooked through. Discard any mussels or clams that do not open.
5. Stir in fresh cilantro and lime juice.
6. Serve immediately.

Number of Serves: 4

Nutritional Info per Serving:

- Calories: 280
- Protein: 35g
- Carbohydrates: 10g
- Fiber: 3g
- Sugars: 4g
- Fat: 10g

Cooking Time: 25 minutes

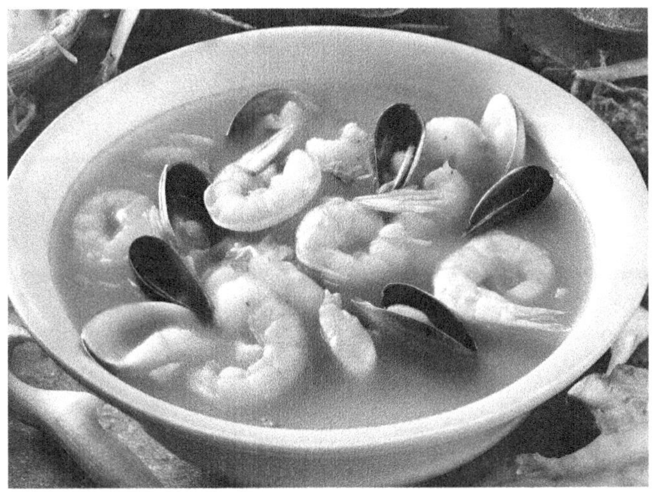

27. Teriyaki Salmon with Broccoli

Ingredients:

- 4 salmon fillets (about 6 oz each)
- 1/4 cup low-sodium soy sauce or tamari
- 2 tablespoons honey or maple syrup
- 1 tablespoon rice vinegar
- 2 cloves garlic, minced
- 1 teaspoon fresh ginger, grated
- 4 cups broccoli florets
- 1 tablespoon sesame oil

Instructions:

1. In a small bowl, whisk together soy sauce or tamari, honey or maple syrup, rice vinegar, garlic, and ginger to make the teriyaki sauce.
2. Place the salmon fillets in a shallow dish and pour half of the teriyaki sauce over them. Let marinate for at least 15 minutes.
3. Preheat the oven to 400°F (200°C).
4. Place the marinated salmon fillets on a baking sheet and bake for 15-20 minutes, or until the salmon is cooked through and flakes easily with a fork.
5. While the salmon is baking, steam the broccoli florets until tender, about 5-7 minutes.
6. Heat sesame oil in a skillet over medium heat. Add the steamed broccoli and stir-fry for 2-3 minutes.
7. Serve the salmon with the remaining teriyaki sauce drizzled over the top and the stir-fried broccoli on the side.

Number of Serves: 4

Nutritional Info per Serving:

- Calories: 350
- Protein: 30g
- Carbohydrates: 15g
- Fiber: 4g
- Sugars: 10g
- Fat: 18g

Cooking Time: 30 minutes

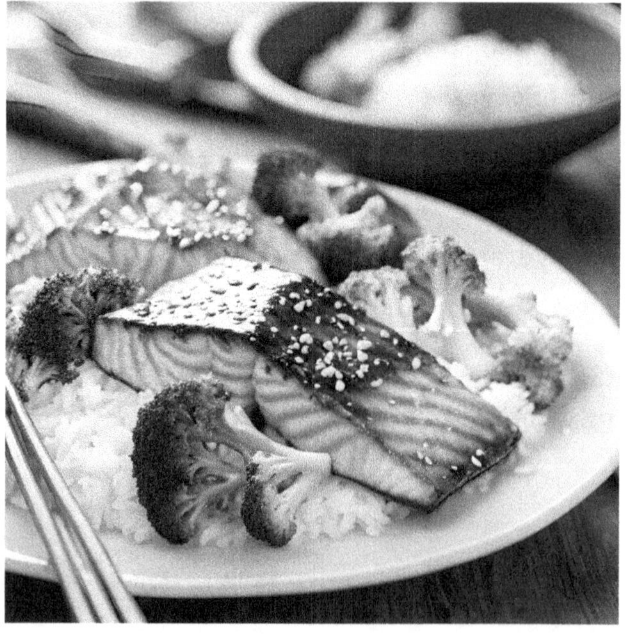

28. Cod en Papillote

Ingredients:

- 4 cod fillets (about 6 oz each)
- 2 zucchinis, thinly sliced
- 1 red bell pepper, thinly sliced
- 1 yellow bell pepper, thinly sliced
- 1 red onion, thinly sliced
- 4 cloves garlic, minced
- 4 tablespoons olive oil
- 4 tablespoons fresh lemon juice
- 2 tablespoons fresh parsley, chopped
- 2 tablespoons fresh thyme, chopped

Instructions:

1. Preheat the oven to 375°F (190°C).
2. Cut four large pieces of parchment paper.
3. Place a cod fillet in the center of each piece of parchment paper.
4. Divide the zucchini, bell peppers, red onion, and garlic evenly among the parchment pieces, placing the vegetables around the fish.
5. Drizzle each fillet and vegetables with 1 tablespoon of olive oil and 1 tablespoon of lemon juice.
6. Sprinkle with fresh parsley and thyme.
7. Fold the parchment paper over the fish and vegetables, crimping the edges to seal and create a packet.
8. Place the packets on a baking sheet and bake for 20-25 minutes, or until the cod is opaque and flakes easily with a fork.
9. Serve immediately.

Number of Serves: 4

Nutritional Info per Serving:

- Calories: 280
- Protein: 30g
- Carbohydrates: 10g
- Fiber: 3g
- Sugars: 5g
- Fat: 14g

Cooking Time: 30 minutes

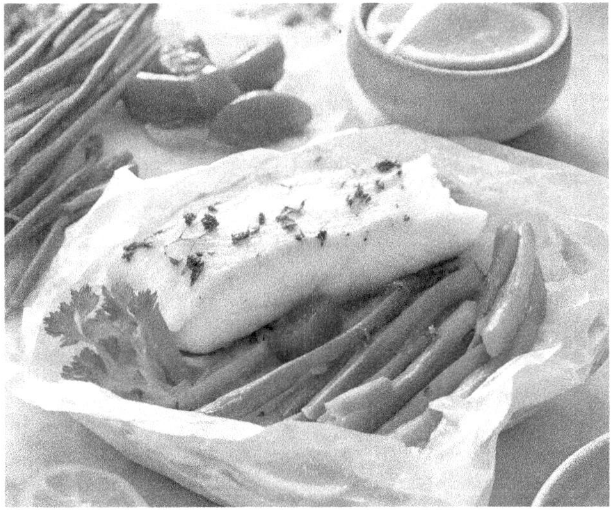

Soup & Stew

1. Jerusalem Artichoke Soup
Ingredients:
- 2 tablespoons olive oil
- 1 onion, chopped
- 3 cloves garlic, minced
- 1 lb (450g) Jerusalem artichokes, peeled and chopped
- 2 cups low-sodium vegetable broth
- 1 cup unsweetened almond milk (or any plant-based milk)
- 1 teaspoon ground turmeric
- 1 teaspoon fresh thyme, chopped
- 1/4 cup fresh parsley, chopped (for garnish)

Instructions:
1. Heat olive oil in a large pot over medium heat.
2. Add onion and garlic, and cook until softened, about 5 minutes.
3. Add chopped Jerusalem artichokes, turmeric, and fresh thyme. Cook for another 2 minutes.
4. Pour in vegetable broth and almond milk. Bring to a boil, then reduce heat and simmer for 20-25 minutes, or until the artichokes are tender.
5. Use an immersion blender to puree the soup until smooth (or transfer to a blender in batches).
6. Serve hot, garnished with fresh parsley.

Number of Serves: 4
Nutritional Info per Serving:
- Calories: 180
- Protein: 3g
- Carbohydrates: 22g
- Fiber: 4g
- Sugars: 4g
- Fat: 9g

Cooking Time: 30 minutes

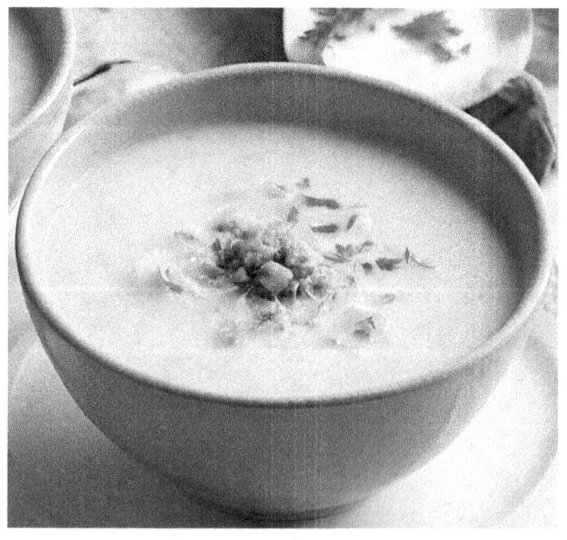

2. Brazilian Fish Stew (Moqueca)

Ingredients:

- 1 lb (450g) white fish fillets (such as cod or halibut), cut into chunks
- 1 tablespoon lime juice
- 2 tablespoons olive oil
- 1 onion, chopped
- 1 red bell pepper, chopped
- 1 yellow bell pepper, chopped
- 3 cloves garlic, minced
- 1 teaspoon ground cumin
- 1 teaspoon paprika
- 1 can (14.5 oz) diced tomatoes
- 1 can (14 oz) coconut milk
- 1/4 cup fresh cilantro, chopped

Instructions:

1. In a bowl, toss the fish chunks with lime juice and set aside.
2. Heat olive oil in a large pot over medium heat.
3. Add onion, red and yellow bell peppers, and garlic. Cook until softened, about 5 minutes.
4. Stir in ground cumin and paprika. Cook for another 2 minutes.
5. Add diced tomatoes and coconut milk. Bring to a simmer.
6. Add the fish chunks and cook for about 10 minutes, or until the fish is cooked through.
7. Stir in fresh cilantro and serve hot.

Number of Serves: 4

Nutritional Info per Serving:

- Calories: 350
- Protein: 30g
- Carbohydrates: 14g
- Fiber: 4g
- Sugars: 6g
- Fat: 20g

Cooking Time: 30 minutes

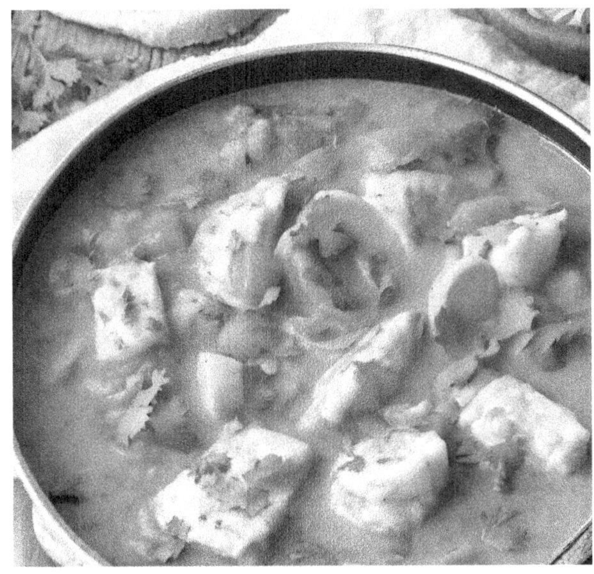

3. Turkish Lentil Soup

Ingredients:

- 2 tablespoons olive oil
- 1 onion, chopped
- 2 cloves garlic, minced
- 1 carrot, chopped
- 1 cup red lentils, rinsed
- 1 teaspoon ground cumin
- 1 teaspoon ground coriander
- 1/2 teaspoon ground turmeric
- 1/4 teaspoon ground paprika
- 4 cups low-sodium vegetable broth
- 1/4 cup fresh parsley, chopped (for garnish)
- 1 lemon, cut into wedges (for serving)

Instructions:

1. Heat olive oil in a large pot over medium heat.
2. Add onion, garlic, and carrot. Cook until softened, about 5 minutes.
3. Stir in red lentils, ground cumin, coriander, turmeric, and paprika. Cook for another 2 minutes.
4. Pour in vegetable broth. Bring to a boil, then reduce heat and simmer for 20-25 minutes, or until the lentils are tender.
5. Use an immersion blender to puree the soup until smooth (or transfer to a blender in batches).
6. Serve hot, garnished with fresh parsley and lemon wedges on the side.

Number of Serves: 4

Nutritional Info per Serving:

- Calories: 220
- Protein: 10g
- Carbohydrates: 30g
- Fiber: 10g
- Sugars: 5g
- Fat: 8g

Cooking Time: 30 minutes

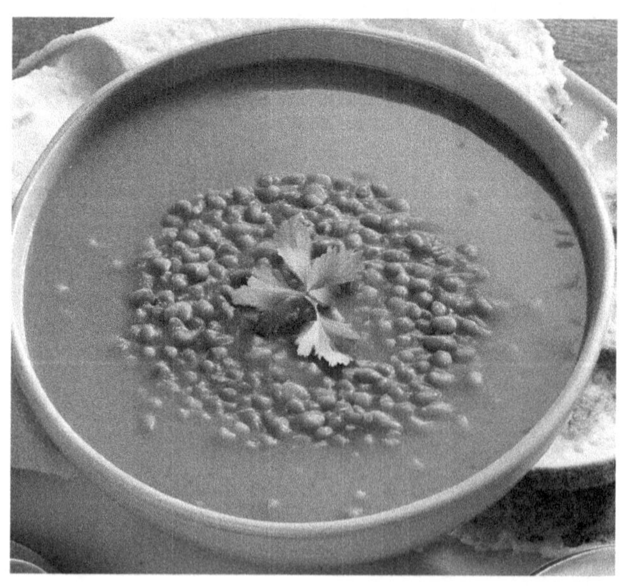

4. Thai Coconut Shrimp Soup

Ingredients:

- 1 tablespoon olive oil
- 1 onion, chopped
- 3 cloves garlic, minced
- 1 tablespoon fresh ginger, grated
- 1 red bell pepper, sliced
- 1 can (14 oz) coconut milk
- 4 cups low-sodium chicken broth
- 1 lb (450g) shrimp, peeled and deveined
- 1 tablespoon fish sauce
- 2 tablespoons fresh lime juice
- 1/4 cup fresh cilantro, chopped

Instructions:

1. Heat olive oil in a large pot over medium heat.
2. Add onion, garlic, ginger, and red bell pepper. Cook until softened, about 5 minutes.
3. Stir in coconut milk and chicken broth. Bring to a simmer.
4. Add shrimp and cook for about 5 minutes, or until shrimp are pink and cooked through.
5. Stir in fish sauce and lime juice.
6. Serve hot, garnished with fresh cilantro.

Number of Serves: 4

Nutritional Info per Serving:

- Calories: 290
- Protein: 20g
- Carbohydrates: 10g
- Fiber: 3g
- Sugars: 4g
- Fat: 18g

Cooking Time: 20 minutes

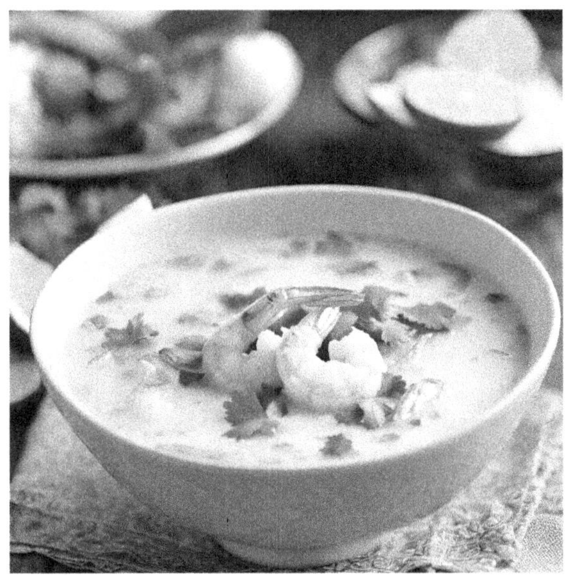

5. Italian Fish Stew

Ingredients:

- 2 tablespoons olive oil
- 1 onion, chopped
- 3 cloves garlic, minced
- 1 fennel bulb, chopped
- 1 can (14.5 oz) diced tomatoes
- 4 cups low-sodium fish or vegetable broth
- 1 lb (450g) white fish fillets (such as cod or haddock), cut into chunks
- 1/2 lb (225g) mussels, cleaned
- 1/2 lb (225g) clams, cleaned
- 1/4 cup fresh parsley, chopped
- 1 tablespoon fresh basil, chopped

Instructions:

1. Heat olive oil in a large pot over medium heat.
2. Add onion, garlic, and fennel. Cook until softened, about 5 minutes.
3. Stir in diced tomatoes and broth. Bring to a simmer.
4. Add the white fish chunks, mussels, and clams. Cover and cook for about 10 minutes, or until the mussels and clams have opened and the fish is cooked through. Discard any mussels or clams that do not open.
5. Stir in fresh parsley and basil.
6. Serve hot.

Number of Serves: 4

Nutritional Info per Serving:

- Calories: 280
- Protein: 30g
- Carbohydrates: 10g
- Fiber: 2g
- Sugars: 4g
- Fat: 12g

Cooking Time: 25 minute

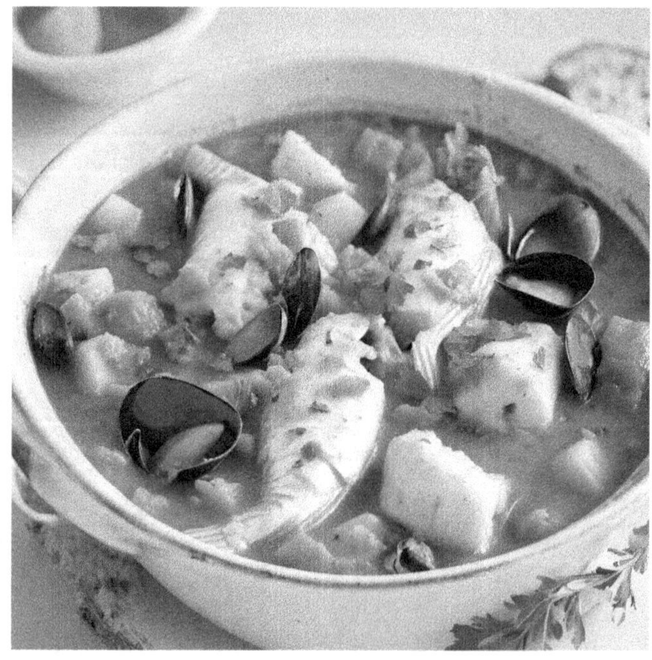

6. Persian Herb Stew (Ghormeh Sabzi)

Ingredients:

- 2 tablespoons olive oil
- 1 onion, chopped
- 3 cloves garlic, minced
- 1 lb (450g) lamb or beef stew meat, cubed
- 1 cup dried kidney beans, soaked overnight and drained
- 2 cups fresh parsley, chopped
- 1 cup fresh cilantro, chopped
- 1 cup fresh chives or green onions, chopped
- 1/4 cup dried fenugreek leaves
- 1 teaspoon turmeric
- 2 dried limes (limoo amani), pierced with a fork
- 4 cups low-sodium vegetable or beef broth
- 1 tablespoon lemon juice

Instructions:

1. Heat olive oil in a large pot over medium heat. Add the onion and garlic and cook until softened, about 5 minutes.
2. Add the meat and turmeric. Cook until browned on all sides, about 10 minutes.
3. Stir in the kidney beans, parsley, cilantro, chives, and dried fenugreek leaves. Cook for another 5 minutes, stirring occasionally.
4. Add the dried limes and broth. Bring to a boil, then reduce heat and simmer for 1.5 to 2 hours, until the meat and beans are tender.
5. Stir in the lemon juice just before serving.
6. Serve hot.

Number of Serves: 6

Nutritional Info per Serving:

- Calories: 300
- Protein: 25g
- Carbohydrates: 25g
- Fiber: 8g
- Sugars: 4g
- Fat: 12g

Cooking Time: 2.5 hours (including simmering time)

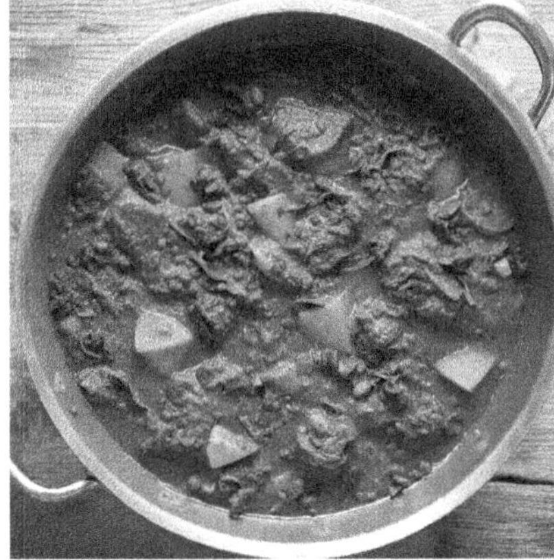

7. Fennel and White Fish Stew

Ingredients:

- 2 tablespoons olive oil
- 1 onion, chopped
- 2 cloves garlic, minced
- 1 fennel bulb, sliced
- 1 can (14.5 oz) diced tomatoes
- 4 cups low-sodium fish or vegetable broth
- 1 lb (450g) white fish fillets (such as cod or haddock), cut into chunks
- 1/4 cup fresh dill, chopped
- 1/4 cup fresh parsley, chopped
- 1 tablespoon lemon juice

Instructions:

1. Heat olive oil in a large pot over medium heat. Add onion, garlic, and fennel. Cook until softened, about 5 minutes.
2. Stir in the diced tomatoes and broth. Bring to a simmer.
3. Add the fish chunks and cook for about 10 minutes, until the fish is cooked through.
4. Stir in fresh dill, parsley, and lemon juice.
5. Serve hot.

Number of Serves: 4

Nutritional Info per Serving:

- Calories: 220
- Protein: 30g
- Carbohydrates: 12g
- Fiber: 4g
- Sugars: 5g
- Fat: 8g

Cooking Time: 25 minutes

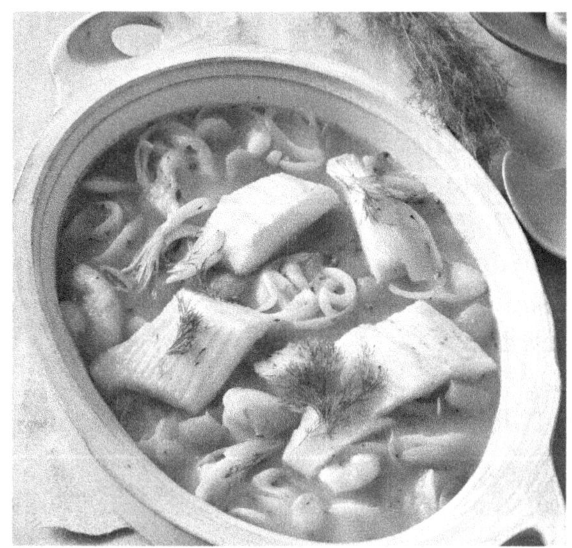

8. Nordic Salmon Soup
Ingredients:
- 2 tablespoons olive oil
- 1 onion, chopped
- 2 carrots, sliced
- 2 celery stalks, sliced
- 1 lb (450g) salmon fillets, cut into chunks
- 4 cups low-sodium fish or vegetable broth
- 1 cup unsweetened almond milk (or any plant-based milk)
- 1/2 teaspoon ground turmeric
- 1/4 cup fresh dill, chopped
- 1 tablespoon lemon juice

Instructions:
1. Heat olive oil in a large pot over medium heat. Add onion, carrots, and celery. Cook until softened, about 5 minutes.
2. Stir in the broth and bring to a simmer.
3. Add the salmon chunks and turmeric. Cook for about 10 minutes, until the salmon is cooked through.
4. Stir in the almond milk, fresh dill, and lemon juice. Cook for an additional 5 minutes.
5. Serve hot.

Number of Serves: 4
Nutritional Info per Serving:
- Calories: 300
- Protein: 28g
- Carbohydrates: 10g
- Fiber: 3g
- Sugars: 4g
- Fat: 16g

Cooking Time: 30 minutes

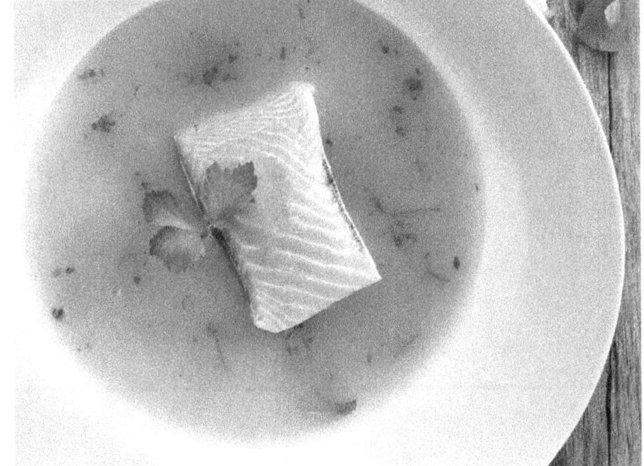

9. Portuguese Kale Soup

Ingredients:

- 2 tablespoons olive oil
- 1 onion, chopped
- 3 cloves garlic, minced
- 1 lb (450g) potatoes, peeled and diced
- 1 can (14.5 oz) diced tomatoes
- 4 cups low-sodium vegetable broth
- 4 cups kale, chopped
- 1 teaspoon smoked paprika
- 1/2 teaspoon ground cumin

Instructions:

1. Heat olive oil in a large pot over medium heat. Add onion and garlic. Cook until softened, about 5 minutes.
2. Add diced potatoes, tomatoes, and vegetable broth. Bring to a boil, then reduce heat and simmer for 15 minutes, or until the potatoes are tender.
3. Stir in the kale, smoked paprika, and ground cumin. Cook for an additional 10 minutes.
4. Serve hot.

Number of Serves: 4

Nutritional Info per Serving:

- Calories: 220
- Protein: 6g
- Carbohydrates: 35g
- Fiber: 8g
- Sugars: 7g
- Fat: 8g

Cooking Time: 30 minutes

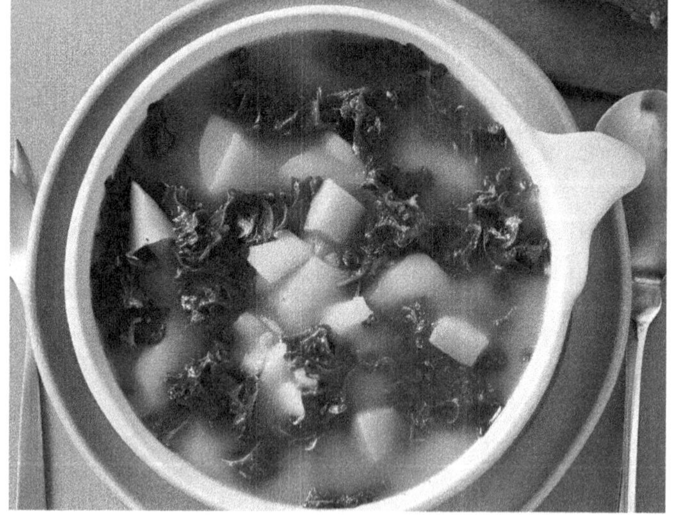

10. Italian White Bean and Spinach Soup

Ingredients:

- 2 tablespoons olive oil
- 1 onion, chopped
- 3 cloves garlic, minced
- 2 carrots, sliced
- 1 can (14.5 oz) diced tomatoes
- 4 cups low-sodium vegetable broth
- 1 can (15 oz) cannellini beans, drained and rinsed
- 4 cups fresh spinach, chopped
- 1 teaspoon dried basil
- 1 teaspoon dried oregano

Instructions:

1. Heat olive oil in a large pot over medium heat. Add onion, garlic, and carrots. Cook until softened, about 5 minutes.
2. Stir in diced tomatoes, vegetable broth, and cannellini beans. Bring to a simmer.
3. Add chopped spinach, dried basil, and oregano. Cook for about 10 minutes, until the spinach is wilted and the soup is heated through.
4. Serve hot.

Number of Serves: 4

Nutritional Info per Serving:

- Calories: 220
- Protein: 8g
- Carbohydrates: 30g
- Fiber: 10g
- Sugars: 6g
- Fat: 8g

Cooking Time: 25 minutes

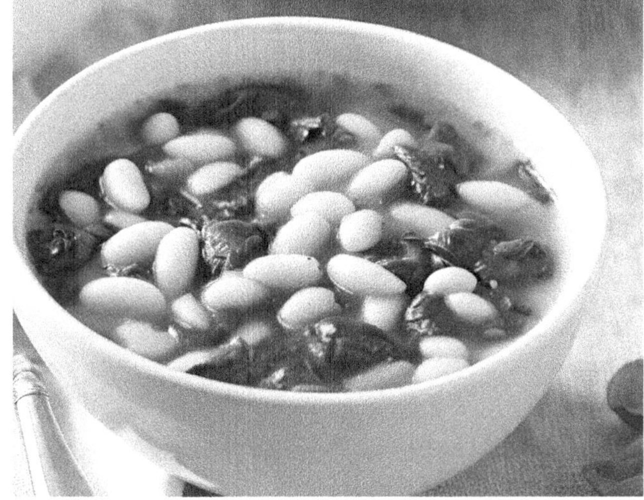

11. Squash and Corn Chowder

Ingredients:

- 2 tablespoons olive oil
- 1 onion, chopped
- 3 cloves garlic, minced
- 1 lb (450g) butternut squash, peeled and diced
- 2 cups corn kernels (fresh or frozen)
- 4 cups low-sodium vegetable broth
- 1 cup unsweetened almond milk (or any plant-based milk)
- 1 teaspoon ground cumin
- 1/4 cup fresh cilantro, chopped (for garnish)

Instructions:

1. Heat olive oil in a large pot over medium heat. Add onion and garlic. Cook until softened, about 5 minutes.
2. Add diced butternut squash, corn, vegetable broth, and ground cumin. Bring to a boil, then reduce heat and simmer for 20 minutes, or until the squash is tender.
3. Stir in the almond milk and cook for an additional 5 minutes.
4. Use an immersion blender to partially blend the soup, leaving some chunks for texture.
5. Serve hot, garnished with fresh cilantro.

Number of Serves: 4

Nutritional Info per Serving:

- Calories: 250
- Protein: 5g
- Carbohydrates: 40g
- Fiber: 8g
- Sugars: 10g
- Fat: 10g

Cooking Time: 30 minutes

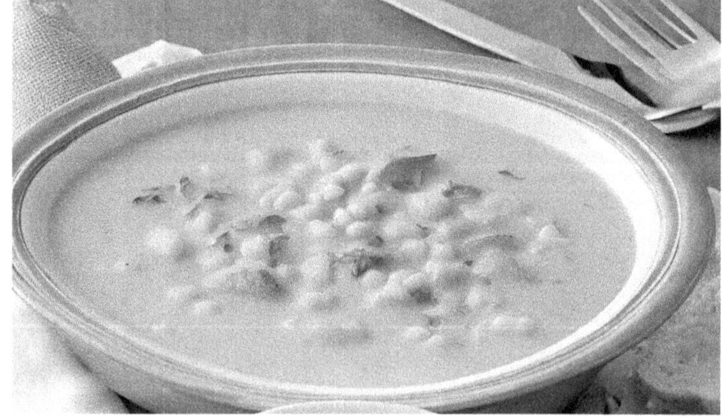

12. Rustic Tomato and Chickpea Stew

Ingredients:

- 2 tablespoons olive oil
- 1 onion, chopped
- 3 cloves garlic, minced
- 2 carrots, sliced
- 1 can (14.5 oz) diced tomatoes
- 1 can (15 oz) chickpeas, drained and rinsed
- 4 cups low-sodium vegetable broth
- 1 teaspoon ground cumin
- 1 teaspoon ground coriander
- 1/2 teaspoon ground paprika
- 1/4 cup fresh parsley, chopped (for garnish)

Instructions:

1. Heat olive oil in a large pot over medium heat. Add onion, garlic, and carrots. Cook until softened, about 5 minutes.
2. Stir in diced tomatoes, chickpeas, vegetable broth, ground cumin, coriander, and paprika. Bring to a simmer.
3. Cook for about 20 minutes, until the carrots are tender and the flavors have melded together.
4. Serve hot, garnished with fresh parsley.

Number of Serves: 4

Nutritional Info per Serving:

- Calories: 220
- Protein: 8g
- Carbohydrates: 35g
- Fiber: 10g
- Sugars: 7g
- Fat: 8g

Cooking Time: 30 minutes

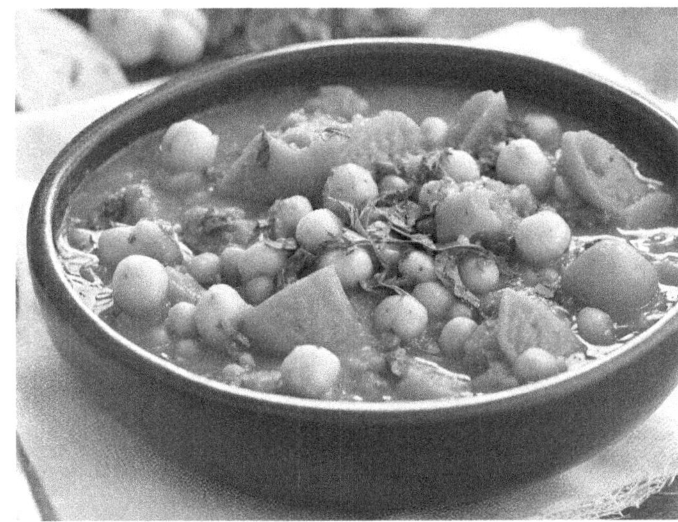

13. Curried Cauliflower Soup

Ingredients:

- 2 tablespoons olive oil
- 1 onion, chopped
- 3 cloves garlic, minced
- 1 head cauliflower, chopped
- 1 tablespoon curry powder
- 1 teaspoon ground turmeric
- 4 cups low-sodium vegetable broth
- 1 cup unsweetened coconut milk
- 1/4 cup fresh cilantro, chopped (for garnish)

Instructions:

1. Heat olive oil in a large pot over medium heat. Add onion and garlic, and cook until softened, about 5 minutes.
2. Add chopped cauliflower, curry powder, and turmeric. Cook for another 2 minutes.
3. Pour in vegetable broth and bring to a boil. Reduce heat and simmer for 20 minutes, or until the cauliflower is tender.
4. Use an immersion blender to puree the soup until smooth (or transfer to a blender in batches).
5. Stir in the coconut milk and cook for an additional 5 minutes.
6. Serve hot, garnished with fresh cilantro.

Number of Serves: 4

Nutritional Info per Serving:

- Calories: 220
- Protein: 4g
- Carbohydrates: 18g
- Fiber: 6g
- Sugars: 6g
- Fat: 16g

Cooking Time: 30 minutes

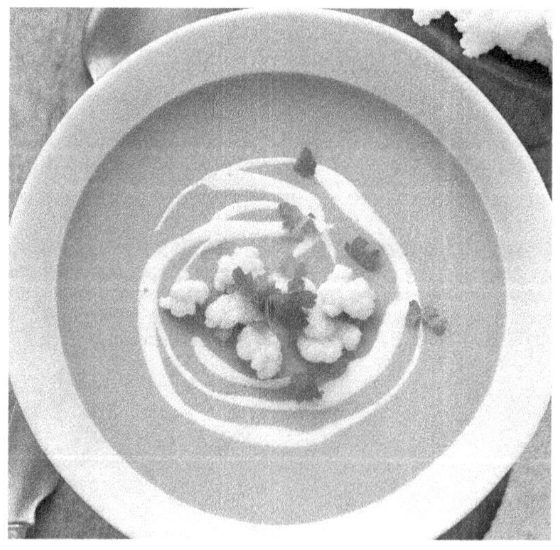

14. Parsnip and Pear Soup

Ingredients:

- 2 tablespoons olive oil
- 1 onion, chopped
- 3 cloves garlic, minced
- 4 parsnips, peeled and chopped
- 2 pears, peeled, cored, and chopped
- 4 cups low-sodium vegetable broth
- 1 teaspoon ground ginger
- 1/2 teaspoon ground nutmeg
- 1/4 cup fresh parsley, chopped (for garnish)

Instructions:

1. Heat olive oil in a large pot over medium heat. Add onion and garlic, and cook until softened, about 5 minutes.
2. Add chopped parsnips and pears. Cook for another 5 minutes.
3. Stir in ground ginger and nutmeg.
4. Pour in vegetable broth and bring to a boil. Reduce heat and simmer for 20-25 minutes, or until the parsnips are tender.
5. Use an immersion blender to puree the soup until smooth (or transfer to a blender in batches).
6. Serve hot, garnished with fresh parsley.

Number of Serves: 4

Nutritional Info per Serving:

- Calories: 210
- Protein: 3g
- Carbohydrates: 34g
- Fiber: 8g
- Sugars: 12g
- Fat: 7g

Cooking Time: 30 minutes

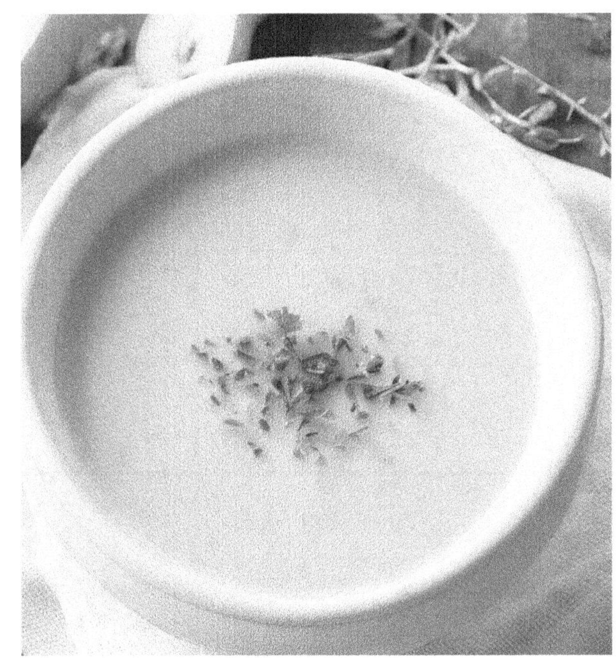

15. Celery Root Soup

Ingredients:

- 2 tablespoons olive oil
- 1 onion, chopped
- 3 cloves garlic, minced
- 1 large celery root (celeriac), peeled and chopped
- 2 potatoes, peeled and chopped
- 4 cups low-sodium vegetable broth
- 1 teaspoon dried thyme
- 1/4 cup fresh chives, chopped (for garnish)

Instructions:

1. Heat olive oil in a large pot over medium heat. Add onion and garlic, and cook until softened, about 5 minutes.
2. Add chopped celery root and potatoes. Cook for another 5 minutes.
3. Stir in dried thyme.
4. Pour in vegetable broth and bring to a boil. Reduce heat and simmer for 20-25 minutes, or until the vegetables are tender.
5. Use an immersion blender to puree the soup until smooth (or transfer to a blender in batches).
6. Serve hot, garnished with fresh chives.

Number of Serves: 4

Nutritional Info per Serving:

- Calories: 200
- Protein: 4g
- Carbohydrates: 35g
- Fiber: 6g
- Sugars: 5g
- Fat: 7g

Cooking Time: 30 minutes

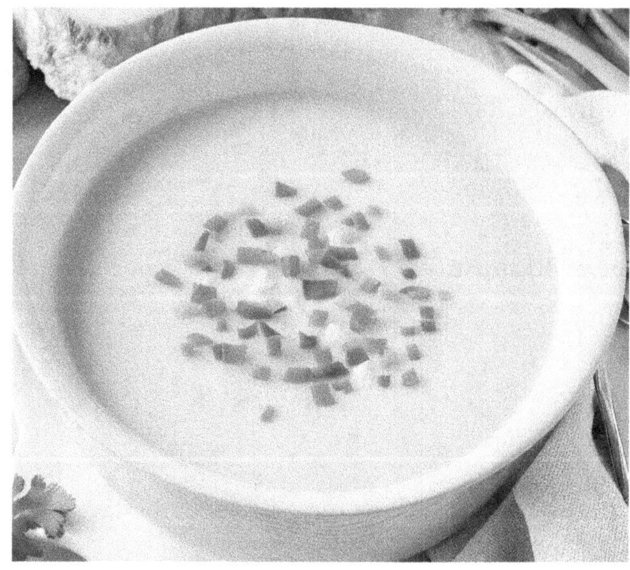

16. Zucchini Basil Soup

Ingredients:

- 2 tablespoons olive oil
- 1 onion, chopped
- 3 cloves garlic, minced
- 4 zucchinis, chopped
- 4 cups low-sodium vegetable broth
- 1 cup fresh basil leaves
- 1/2 cup unsweetened almond milk (or any plant-based milk)
- 1/4 cup fresh basil, chopped (for garnish)

Instructions:

1. Heat olive oil in a large pot over medium heat. Add onion and garlic, and cook until softened, about 5 minutes.
2. Add chopped zucchinis and cook for another 5 minutes.
3. Pour in vegetable broth and bring to a boil. Reduce heat and simmer for 15-20 minutes, or until the zucchinis are tender.
4. Stir in the fresh basil leaves.
5. Use an immersion blender to puree the soup until smooth (or transfer to a blender in batches).
6. Stir in the almond milk and cook for an additional 5 minutes.
7. Serve hot, garnished with chopped basil.

Number of Serves: 4

Nutritional Info per Serving:

- Calories: 180
- Protein: 4g
- Carbohydrates: 18g
- Fiber: 4g
- Sugars: 8g
- Fat: 12g

Cooking Time: 30 minutes

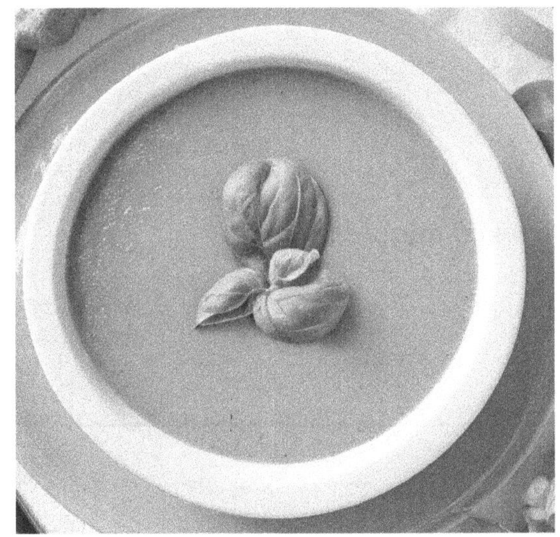

17. Leek and Potato Soup
Ingredients:
- 2 tablespoons olive oil
- 3 leeks, white and light green parts only, sliced
- 3 cloves garlic, minced
- 4 potatoes, peeled and chopped
- 4 cups low-sodium vegetable broth
- 1 cup unsweetened almond milk (or any plant-based milk)
- 1/4 teaspoon ground nutmeg
- 1/4 cup fresh chives, chopped (for garnish)

Instructions:
1. Heat olive oil in a large pot over medium heat. Add sliced leeks and garlic, and cook until softened, about 5 minutes.
2. Add chopped potatoes and cook for another 5 minutes.
3. Pour in vegetable broth and bring to a boil. Reduce heat and simmer for 20-25 minutes, or until the potatoes are tender.
4. Use an immersion blender to puree the soup until smooth (or transfer to a blender in batches).
5. Stir in the almond milk and ground nutmeg. Cook for an additional 5 minutes.
6. Serve hot, garnished with fresh chives.

Number of Serves: 4
Nutritional Info per Serving:
- Calories: 220
- Protein: 4g
- Carbohydrates: 34g
- Fiber: 5g
- Sugars: 5g
- Fat: 9g

Cooking Time: 30 minutes

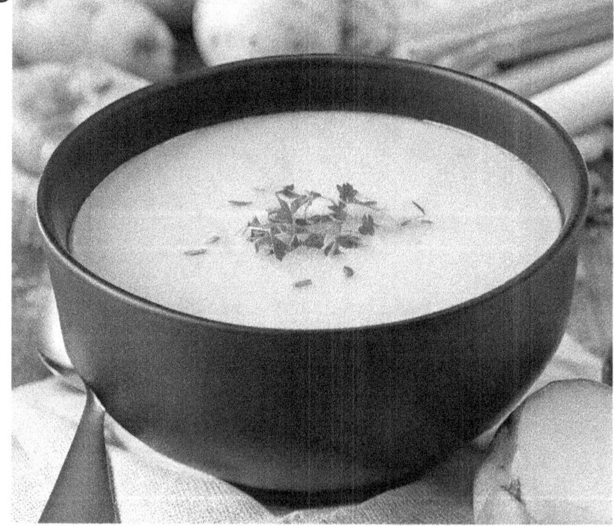

18. Mushroom and Tarragon Soup

Ingredients:

- 2 tablespoons olive oil
- 1 onion, chopped
- 3 cloves garlic, minced
- 1 lb (450g) mushrooms, sliced
- 4 cups low-sodium vegetable broth
- 1 cup unsweetened almond milk (or any plant-based milk)
- 1 teaspoon dried tarragon
- 1/4 cup fresh parsley, chopped (for garnish)

Instructions:

1. Heat olive oil in a large pot over medium heat. Add onion and garlic, and cook until softened, about 5 minutes.
2. Add sliced mushrooms and cook until they release their juices and become tender, about 10 minutes.
3. Stir in dried tarragon.
4. Pour in vegetable broth and bring to a boil. Reduce heat and simmer for 15 minutes.
5. Use an immersion blender to puree the soup until smooth (or transfer to a blender in batches).
6. Stir in the almond milk and cook for an additional 5 minutes.
7. Serve hot, garnished with fresh parsley.

Number of Serves: 4

Nutritional Info per Serving:

- Calories: 200
- Protein: 6g
- Carbohydrates: 15g
- Fiber: 4g
- Sugars: 6g
- Fat: 14g

Cooking Time: 30 minutes

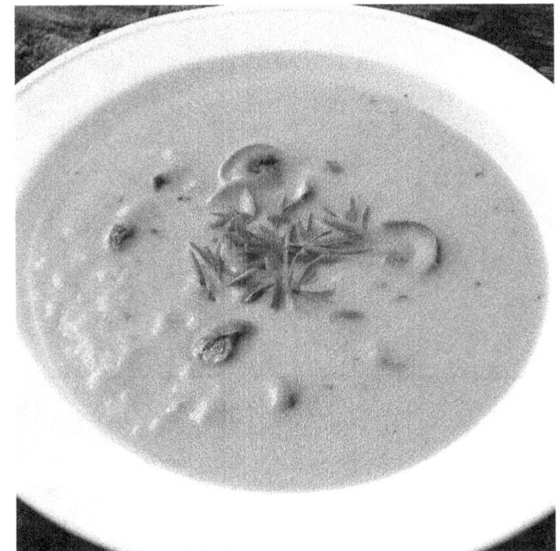

19. Broccoli and Arugula Soup

Ingredients:

- 2 tablespoons olive oil
- 1 onion, chopped
- 3 cloves garlic, minced
- 4 cups broccoli florets
- 4 cups low-sodium vegetable broth
- 2 cups arugula, packed
- 1 cup unsweetened almond milk (or any plant-based milk)
- 1 teaspoon ground turmeric
- 1/4 cup fresh parsley, chopped (for garnish)

Instructions:

1. Heat olive oil in a large pot over medium heat. Add onion and garlic, and cook until softened, about 5 minutes.
2. Add broccoli florets and turmeric. Cook for another 3 minutes.
3. Pour in vegetable broth and bring to a boil. Reduce heat and simmer for 15-20 minutes, or until the broccoli is tender.
4. Stir in the arugula and cook for another 2 minutes.
5. Use an immersion blender to puree the soup until smooth (or transfer to a blender in batches).
6. Stir in the almond milk and cook for an additional 5 minutes.
7. Serve hot, garnished with fresh parsley.

Number of Serves: 4

Nutritional Info per Serving:

- Calories: 180
- Protein: 6g
- Carbohydrates: 18g
- Fiber: 6g
- Sugars: 5g
- Fat: 10g

Cooking Time: 30 minutes

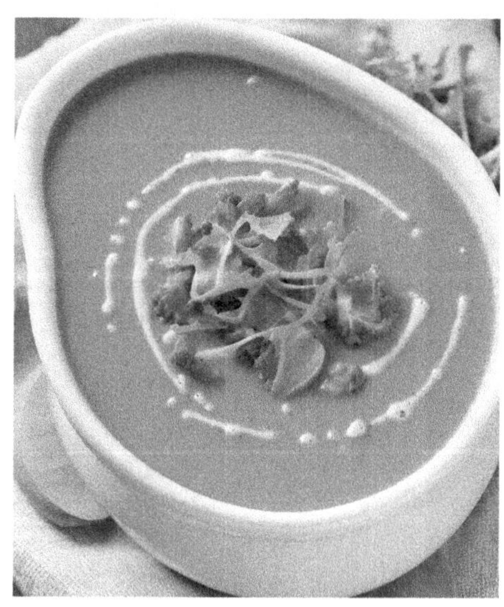

20. Kale and White Bean Soup

Ingredients:
- 2 tablespoons olive oil
- 1 onion, chopped
- 3 cloves garlic, minced
- 4 cups kale, chopped
- 1 can (15 oz) cannellini beans, drained and rinsed
- 4 cups low-sodium vegetable broth
- 1 can (14.5 oz) diced tomatoes
- 1 teaspoon dried thyme
- 1 teaspoon dried basil
- 1/4 cup fresh parsley, chopped (for garnish)

Instructions:
1. Heat olive oil in a large pot over medium heat. Add onion and garlic, and cook until softened, about 5 minutes.
2. Stir in chopped kale and cook until wilted, about 5 minutes.
3. Add cannellini beans, diced tomatoes, vegetable broth, thyme, and basil. Bring to a boil.
4. Reduce heat and simmer for 20 minutes, or until the flavors have melded together.
5. Serve hot, garnished with fresh parsley.

Number of Serves: 4

Nutritional Info per Serving:
- Calories: 220
- Protein: 8g
- Carbohydrates: 30g
- Fiber: 8g
- Sugars: 6g
- Fat: 8g

Cooking Time: 30 minutes

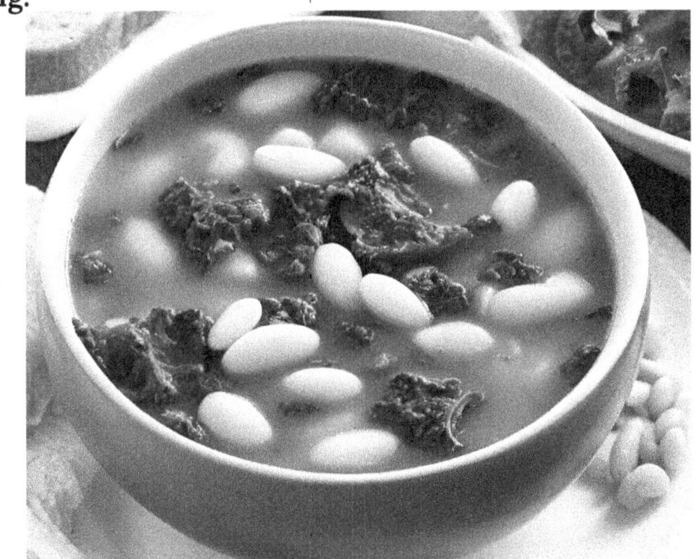

21. Sweet Potato and Coconut Soup

Ingredients:

- 2 tablespoons olive oil
- 1 onion, chopped
- 3 cloves garlic, minced
- 1 tablespoon fresh ginger, grated
- 4 cups sweet potatoes, peeled and chopped
- 4 cups low-sodium vegetable broth
- 1 can (14 oz) coconut milk
- 1 teaspoon ground cumin
- 1/2 teaspoon ground coriander
- 1/4 cup fresh cilantro, chopped (for garnish)

Instructions:

1. Heat olive oil in a large pot over medium heat. Add onion, garlic, and ginger, and cook until softened, about 5 minutes.
2. Add chopped sweet potatoes, cumin, and coriander. Cook for another 3 minutes.
3. Pour in vegetable broth and bring to a boil. Reduce heat and simmer for 20-25 minutes, or until the sweet potatoes are tender.
4. Use an immersion blender to puree the soup until smooth (or transfer to a blender in batches).
5. Stir in the coconut milk and cook for an additional 5 minutes.
6. Serve hot, garnished with fresh cilantro.

Number of Serves: 4

Nutritional Info per Serving:

- Calories: 280
- Protein: 4g
- Carbohydrates: 34g
- Fiber: 6g
- Sugars: 8g
- Fat: 16g

Cooking Time: 30 minutes

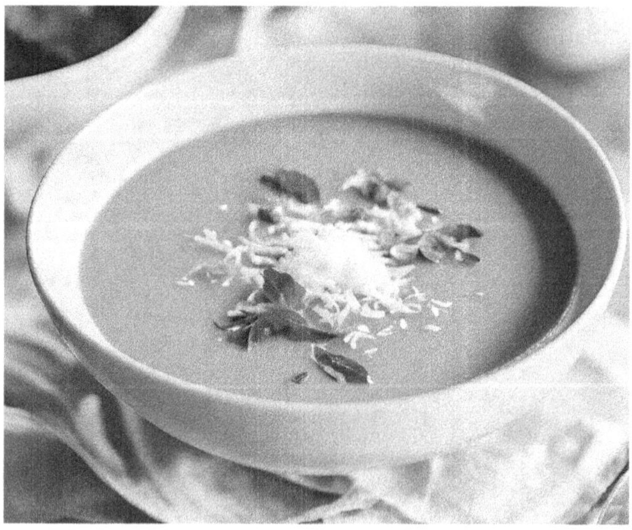

Snacks & Desserts

1. Roasted Chickpeas

Ingredients:

- 1 can (15 oz) chickpeas, drained and rinsed
- 1 tablespoon olive oil
- 1 teaspoon ground cumin
- 1 teaspoon smoked paprika
- 1/2 teaspoon garlic powder

Instructions:

1. Preheat the oven to 400°F (200°C).
2. Pat the chickpeas dry with a paper towel.
3. In a bowl, toss the chickpeas with olive oil, cumin, smoked paprika, and garlic powder.
4. Spread the chickpeas on a baking sheet in a single layer.
5. Roast for 25-30 minutes, stirring halfway through, until the chickpeas are golden and crispy.
6. Let cool slightly before serving.

Number of Serves: 4

Nutritional Info per Serving:

- Calories: 150
- Protein: 6g
- Carbohydrates: 18g
- Fiber: 5g
- Sugars: 1g
- Fat: 7g

Cooking Time: 30 minutes

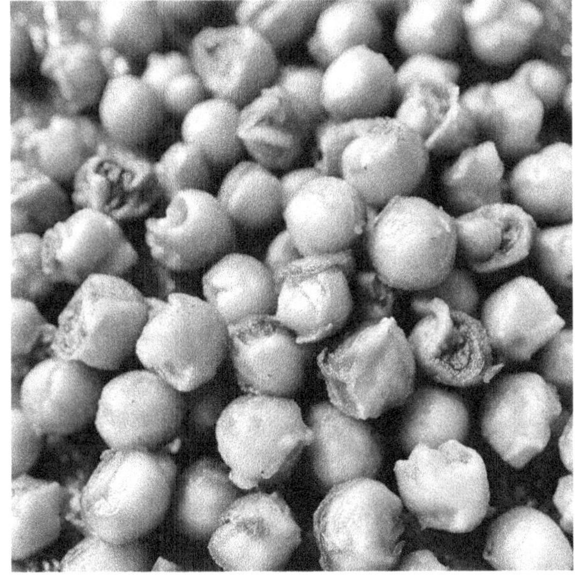

2. Cucumber and Mint Rolls

Ingredients:

- 1 large cucumber, thinly sliced lengthwise
- 1/2 cup hummus
- 1/4 cup fresh mint leaves
- 1/4 cup shredded carrots

Instructions:

1. Lay the cucumber slices flat on a cutting board.
2. Spread a thin layer of hummus over each cucumber slice.
3. Place a few mint leaves and some shredded carrots on one end of each cucumber slice.
4. Roll up the cucumber slices tightly and secure with a toothpick if needed.
5. Serve immediately.

Number of Serves: 4

Nutritional Info per Serving:

- Calories: 70
- Protein: 2g
- Carbohydrates: 8g
- Fiber: 2g
- Sugars: 2g
- Fat: 3g

Cooking Time: 10 minutes

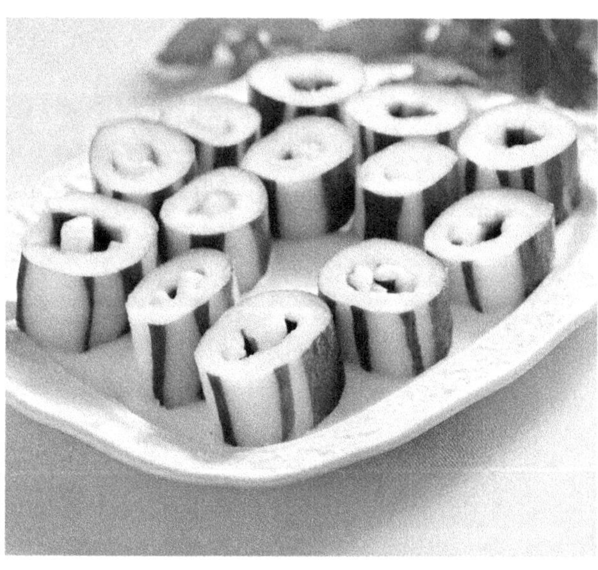

3. Zucchini and Flaxseed Crackers

Ingredients:

- 1 large zucchini, grated
- 1/2 cup ground flaxseed
- 1/4 cup nutritional yeast
- 1 teaspoon dried oregano
- 1 teaspoon garlic powder
- 1/2 teaspoon onion powder

Instructions:

1. Preheat the oven to 350°F (175°C).
2. Place the grated zucchini in a clean kitchen towel and squeeze out the excess moisture.
3. In a bowl, combine zucchini, ground flaxseed, nutritional yeast, oregano, garlic powder, and onion powder. Mix well.
4. Spread the mixture evenly on a parchment-lined baking sheet.
5. Bake for 20-25 minutes, or until the edges are golden and the mixture is firm.
6. Let cool, then cut into cracker-sized pieces.
7. Serve immediately or store in an airtight container.

Number of Serves: 4

Nutritional Info per Serving:

- Calories: 90
- Protein: 4g
- Carbohydrates: 8g
- Fiber: 5g
- Sugars: 2g
- Fat: 5g

Cooking Time: 25 minutes

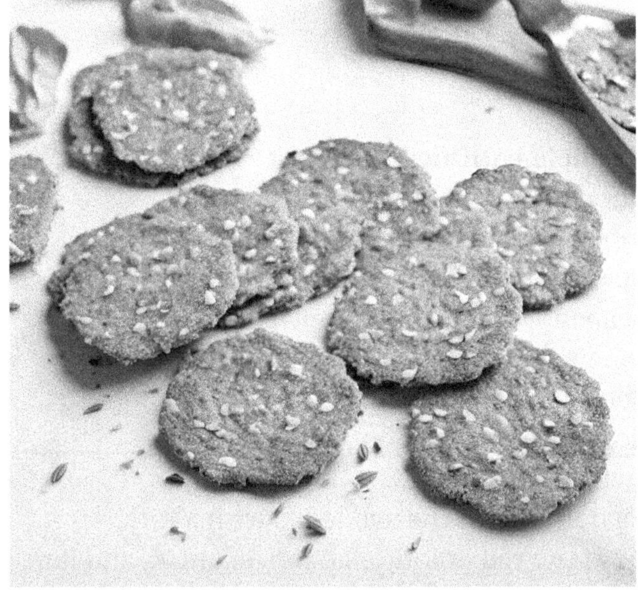

4. Spiced Nuts

Ingredients:

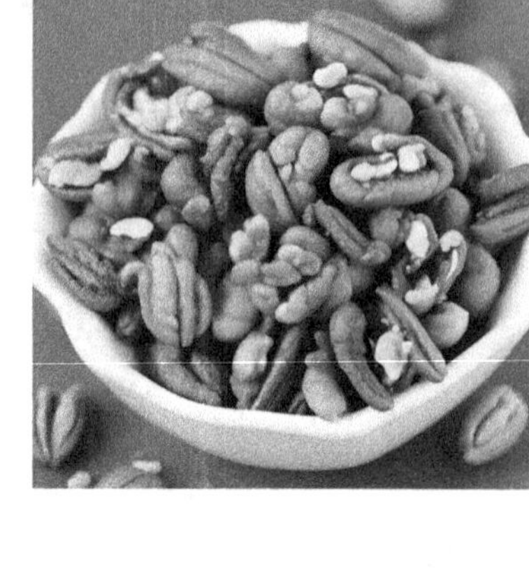

- 1 cup almonds
- 1 cup cashews
- 1 cup walnuts
- 2 tablespoons olive oil
- 1 teaspoon ground cumin
- 1 teaspoon smoked paprika
- 1/2 teaspoon ground cinnamon

Instructions:

1. Preheat the oven to 350°F (175°C).
2. In a bowl, mix the nuts with olive oil, cumin, smoked paprika, and cinnamon until evenly coated.
3. Spread the nuts on a baking sheet in a single layer.
4. Bake for 15-20 minutes, stirring halfway through, until the nuts are golden and fragrant.
5. Let cool completely before serving.

Number of Serves: 8

Nutritional Info per Serving:

- Calories: 200 Protein: 5g Carbohydrates: 8g Fiber: 3g   Sugars: 1g Fat: 18g

Cooking Time: 20 minutes

5. Guacamole with Jicama Sticks

Ingredients:

- 2 ripe avocados, peeled and pitted
- 1 small red onion, finely chopped
- 1 jalapeño, seeded and finely chopped
- 1/4 cup fresh cilantro, chopped
- 2 tablespoons lime juice
- 1 jicama, peeled and cut into sticks

Instructions:

1. In a bowl, mash the avocados with a fork.
2. Stir in the red onion, jalapeño, cilantro, and lime juice until well combined.
3. Serve the guacamole with jicama sticks.

Number of Serves: 4

Nutritional Info per Serving:

- Calories: 170 Protein: 2g Carbohydrates: 14g Fiber: 8g   Sugars: 2g   Fat: 13g

Cooking Time: 10 minutes

6. Pineapple Carpaccio

Ingredients:

- 1 fresh pineapple, peeled and thinly sliced
- 1 tablespoon lime juice
- 1 tablespoon honey or maple syrup
- 1/4 cup fresh mint leaves, chopped

Instructions:

1. Arrange the pineapple slices on a serving platter.
2. Drizzle with lime juice and honey or maple syrup.
3. Sprinkle with fresh mint leaves.
4. Serve immediately.

Number of Serves: 4

Nutritional Info per Serving:

- Calories: 90 Protein: 1g Carbohydrates: 22g Fiber: 2g Sugars: 18g Fat: 0g

Cooking Time: 10 minutes

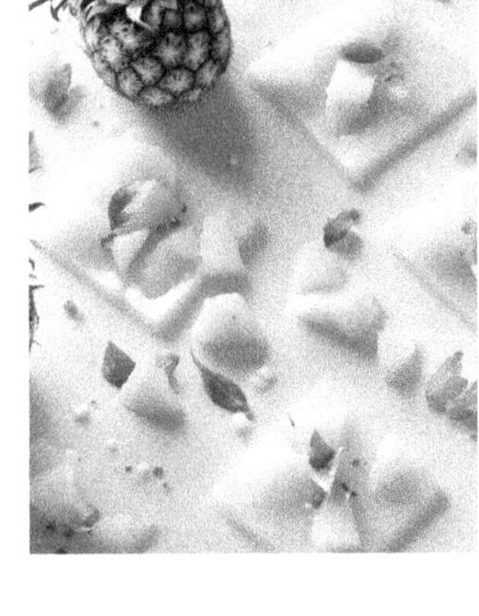

7. Pumpkin Spice Mousse

Ingredients:

- 1 cup pumpkin puree
- 1/2 cup unsweetened coconut cream
- 2 tablespoons maple syrup
- 1 teaspoon ground cinnamon
- 1/2 teaspoon ground nutmeg
- 1/2 teaspoon ground ginger

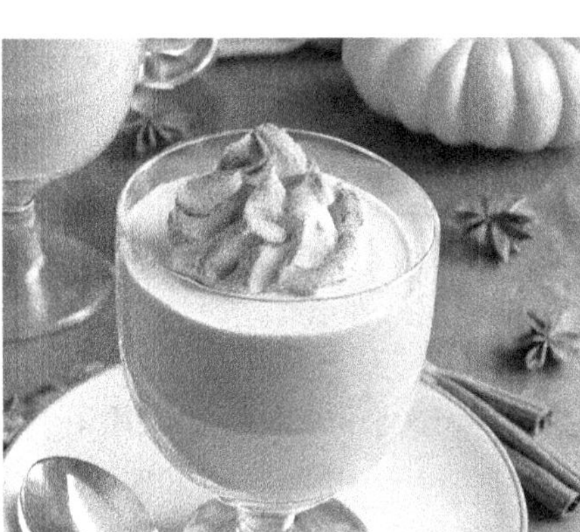

Instructions:

1. In a bowl, whisk together pumpkin puree, coconut cream, maple syrup, cinnamon, nutmeg, and ginger until smooth.
2. Spoon the mixture into serving dishes.
3. Chill in the refrigerator for at least 1 hour before serving.

Number of Serves: 4

Nutritional Info per Serving:

- Calories: 120
- Protein: 1g
- Carbohydrates: 16g
- Fiber: 3g
- Sugars: 10g
- Fat: 6g

Cooking Time: 10 minutes (plus chilling time)

8. Almond and Apricot Bars

Ingredients:

- 1 cup almonds
- 1 cup dried apricots
- 1/2 cup unsweetened shredded coconut
- 2 tablespoons honey or maple syrup
- 1 teaspoon vanilla extract

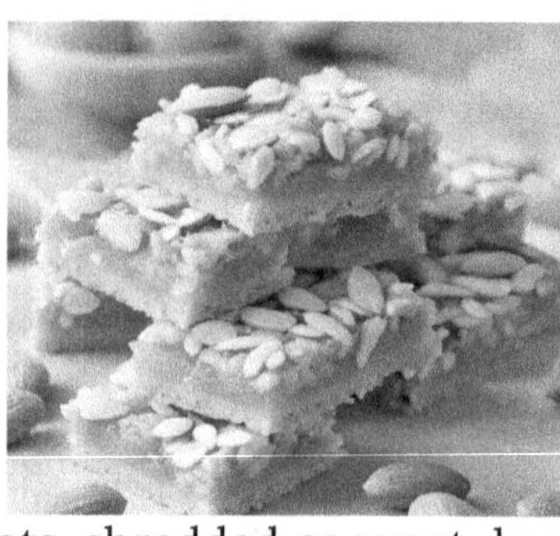

Instructions:

1. In a food processor, combine almonds, dried apricots, shredded coconut, honey or maple syrup, and vanilla extract. Process until the mixture is well combined and sticky.
2. Press the mixture firmly into a parchment-lined baking dish.
3. Chill in the refrigerator for at least 1 hour.
4. Cut into bars and serve.

Number of Serves: 8

Nutritional Info per Serving:

Calories: 180 Protein: 4g Carbohydrates: 20g Fiber: 4g Sugars: 14g Fat: 10g

Cooking Time: 10 minutes (plus chilling time)

9. Watermelon Pizza

Ingredients:

- 1 large watermelon, cut into 1-inch thick rounds
- 1 cup Greek yogurt
- 1/2 cup mixed berries (blueberries, raspberries, strawberries)
- 1/4 cup unsweetened shredded coconut
- 1 tablespoon honey or maple syrup

Instructions:

1. Spread a layer of Greek yogurt over each watermelon round.
2. Top with mixed berries and shredded coconut.
3. Drizzle with honey or maple syrup.
4. Cut into wedges and serve immediately.

Number of Serves: 8

Nutritional Info per Serving:

- Calories: 70
- Protein: 3g
- Carbohydrates: 14g
- Fiber: 2g
- Sugars: 11g
- Fat: 2g

Cooking Time: 10 minutes

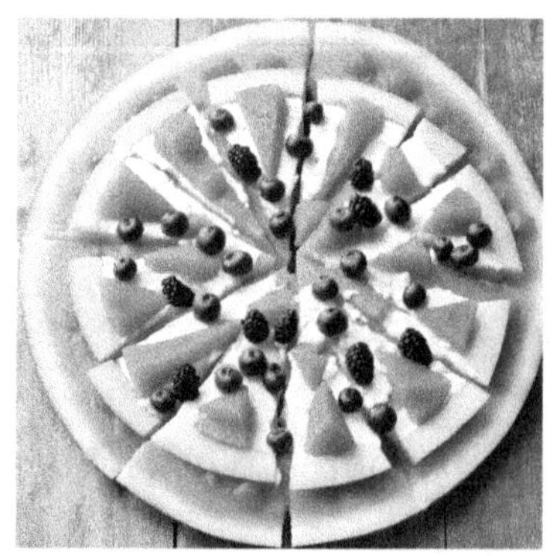

10-WEEK MEAL PLAN

Week 1

Day 1:
- Breakfast: Roasted Chickpeas
- Lunch: Grilled Chicken with Avocado Salsa
- Dinner: Grilled Salmon with Lemon and Dill

Day 2:
- Breakfast: Cucumber and Mint Rolls
- Lunch: Chicken and Quinoa Salad
- Dinner: Spicy Seafood Soup

Day 3:
- Breakfast: Zucchini and Flaxseed Crackers
- Lunch: Shrimp Stir-Fry with Vegetables
- Dinner: Turmeric Chicken Soup

Day 4:
- Breakfast: Spiced Nuts
- Lunch: Baked Cod with Olive Tapenade
- Dinner: Chicken Tikka Masala with Almond Milk

Day 5:
- Breakfast: Guacamole with Jicama Sticks
- Lunch: Seared Tuna Steak with Avocado Salsa
- Dinner: Broccoli and Arugula Soup

Day 6:
- Breakfast: Pineapple Carpaccio
- Lunch: Roasted Chicken Drumsticks with Herbs
- Dinner: Brazilian Fish Stew

Day 7:
- Breakfast: Pumpkin Spice Mousse
- Lunch: Grilled Mahi-Mahi with Pineapple Salsa
- Dinner: Persian Herb Stew (Ghormeh Sabzi)

Week 2

Day 1:
- Breakfast: Almond and Apricot Bars
- Lunch: Chicken and Spinach Stew
- Dinner: Italian Fish Stew

Day 2:
- Breakfast: Watermelon Pizza
- Lunch: Kale and White Bean Soup
- Dinner: Moroccan Chicken Stew

Day 3:

- Breakfast: Turmeric Latte
- Lunch: Grilled Octopus with Olive Oil and Lemon
- Dinner: Steamed Fish with Ginger and Scallions

Day 4:

- Breakfast: Buckwheat Pancakes
- Lunch: Spinach and Walnut Stuffed Chicken
- Dinner: Sweet Potato and Coconut Soup

Day 5:

- Breakfast: Oatmeal with Berries
- Lunch: Herb-Crusted Halibut
- Dinner: Zucchini Basil Soup

Day 6:

- Breakfast: Mixed Berry Salad
- Lunch: One-Pan Harissa Chicken
- Dinner: Curried Cauliflower Soup

Day 7:

- Breakfast: Sautéed Tempeh
- Lunch: Thai Coconut Shrimp Soup
- Dinner: Celery Root Soup

Week 3

Day 1:

- Breakfast: Mango and Spinach Smoothie
- Lunch: Chicken and Mango Salad
- Dinner: Leek and Potato Soup

Day 2:

- Breakfast: Pumpkin Porridge
- Lunch: Prawn Cocktail with Avocado
- Dinner: Mushroom and Tarragon Soup

Day 3:

- Breakfast: Banana Almond Smoothie
- Lunch: Baked Lemon and Herb Chicken
- Dinner: Fennel and White Fish Stew

Day 4:

- Breakfast: Savory Quinoa Bowl
- Lunch: Salmon and Quinoa Salad
- Dinner: Squash and Corn Chowder

Day 5:
- Breakfast: Pea Protein Shake
- Lunch: Tilapia with Mango Salsa
- Dinner: Rustic Tomato and Chickpea Stew

Day 6:
- Breakfast: Almond Butter and Pear Toast
- Lunch: Clam Soup with Vegetables
- Dinner: Portuguese Kale Soup

Day 7:
- Breakfast: Flaxseed Porridge
- Lunch: Baked Trout with Almonds
- Dinner: Italian White Bean and Spinach Soup

Week 4

Day 1:
- Breakfast: Roasted Beetroot Salad
- Lunch: Teriyaki Salmon with Broccoli
- Dinner: Parsnip and Pear Soup

Day 2:
- Breakfast: Zucchini Muffins
- Lunch: Scallop Carpaccio with Citrus Vinaigrette
- Dinner: Turkish Lentil Soup

Day 3:
- Breakfast: Kale Smoothie
- Lunch: Chicken Tenders with Paleo Coating
- Dinner: Ceviche with Citrus and Cilantro

Day 4:
- Breakfast: Mixed Berry Salad
- Lunch: Herbed Chicken and Veggie Soup
- Dinner: Persian Herb Stew (Ghormeh Sabzi)

Day 5:
- Breakfast: Mango and Spinach Smoothie
- Lunch: Baked Lemon Sole
- Dinner: Italian White Bean and Spinach Soup

Day 6:
- Breakfast: Pumpkin Spice Mousse
- Lunch: Grilled Mahi-Mahi with Pineapple Salsa
- Dinner: Fennel and White Fish Stew

Day 7:

- Breakfast: Almond and Apricot Bars
- Lunch: Grilled Octopus with Olive Oil and Lemon
- Dinner: Leek and Potato Soup

Week 5

Day 1:

- Breakfast: Pineapple Carpaccio
- Lunch: Chicken and Mango Salad
- Dinner: Squash and Corn Chowder

Day 2:

- Breakfast: Watermelon Pizza
- Lunch: Moroccan Chicken Stew
- Dinner: Celery Root Soup

Day 3:

- Breakfast: Turmeric Latte
- Lunch: Spinach and Walnut Stuffed Chicken
- Dinner: Sweet Potato and Coconut Soup

Day 4:

- Breakfast: Buckwheat Pancakes
- Lunch: Prawn Cocktail with Avocado
- Dinner: Mushroom and Tarragon Soup

Day 5:

- Breakfast: Oatmeal with Berries
- Lunch: Herb-Crusted Halibut
- Dinner: Zucchini Basil Soup

Day 6:

- Breakfast: Mixed Berry Salad
- Lunch: One-Pan Harissa Chicken
- Dinner: Curried Cauliflower Soup

Day 7:

- Breakfast: Sautéed Tempeh
- Lunch: Thai Coconut Shrimp Soup
- Dinner: Broccoli and Arugula Soup

Week 6

Day 1:

- Breakfast: Cucumber and Lime Chilled Soup
- Lunch: Chicken and Quinoa Salad
- Dinner: Grilled Salmon with Lemon and Dill

Day 2:
- Breakfast: Walnut and Pear Baked Oatmeal
- Lunch: Shrimp Stir-Fry with Vegetables
- Dinner: Turmeric Chicken Soup

Day 3:
- Breakfast: Matcha Green Tea
- Lunch: Baked Cod with Olive Tapenade
- Dinner: Chicken Tikka Masala with Almond Milk

Day 4:
- Breakfast: Kale and Avocado Wrap
- Lunch: Seared Tuna Steak with Avocado Salsa
- Dinner: Broccoli and Arugula Soup

Day 5:
- Breakfast: Spinach and Mushroom Crepes
- Lunch: Roasted Chicken Drumsticks with Herbs
- Dinner: Brazilian Fish Stew

Day 6:
- Breakfast: Quinoa and Chia Porridge
- Lunch: Grilled Mahi-Mahi with Pineapple Salsa
- Dinner: Persian Herb Stew (Ghormeh Sabzi)

Day 7:
- Breakfast: Fruit Salad
- Lunch: Baked Lemon and Herb Chicken
- Dinner: Italian Fish Stew

Week 7

Day 1:
- Breakfast: Amaranth Porridge
- Lunch: Moroccan Chicken Stew
- Dinner: Steamed Fish with Ginger and Scallions

Day 2:
- Breakfast: Turmeric Latte
- Lunch: One-Pan Harissa Chicken
- Dinner: Sweet Potato and Coconut Soup

Day 3:
- Breakfast: Buckwheat Pancakes
- Lunch: Herb-Crusted Halibut
- Dinner: Zucchini Basil Soup

Day 4:
- Breakfast: Oatmeal with Berries
- Lunch: Prawn Cocktail with Avocado
- Dinner: Mushroom and Tarragon Soup

Day 5:
- Breakfast: Mixed Berry Salad
- Lunch: Grilled Octopus with Olive Oil and Lemon
- Dinner: Celery Root Soup

Day 6:
- Breakfast: Sautéed Tempeh
- Lunch: Spinach and Walnut Stuffed Chicken
- Dinner: Curried Cauliflower Soup

Day 7:
- Breakfast: Mango and Spinach Smoothie
- Lunch: Baked Lemon Sole
- Dinner: Leek and Potato Soup

Week 8

Day 1:
- Breakfast: Pumpkin Porridge
- Lunch: Baked Trout with Almonds
- Dinner: Italian White Bean and Spinach Soup

Day 2:
- Breakfast: Banana Almond Smoothie
- Lunch: Tilapia with Mango Salsa
- Dinner: Rustic Tomato and Chickpea Stew

Day 3:
- Breakfast: Savory Quinoa Bowl
- Lunch: Clam Soup with Vegetables
- Dinner: Portuguese Kale Soup

Day 4:
- Breakfast: Pea Protein Shake
- Lunch: Thai Coconut Shrimp Soup
- Dinner: Fennel and White Fish Stew

Day 5:
- Breakfast: Almond Butter and Pear Toast
- Lunch: Grilled Sardines with Herbs
- Dinner: Broccoli and Arugula Soup

Day 6:
- Breakfast: Flaxseed Porridge
- Lunch: Chicken and Mango Salad
- Dinner: Squash and Corn Chowder

Day 7:
- Breakfast: Roasted Beetroot Salad
- Lunch: Teriyaki Salmon with Broccoli
- Dinner: Parsnip and Pear Soup

Week 9

Day 1:
- Breakfast: Zucchini Muffins
- Lunch: Scallop Carpaccio with Citrus Vinaigrette
- Dinner: Turkish Lentil Soup

Day 2:
- Breakfast: Kale Smoothie
- Lunch: Chicken Tenders with Paleo Coating
- Dinner: Ceviche with Citrus and Cilantro

Day 3:
- Breakfast: Mixed Berry Salad
- Lunch: Herbed Chicken and Veggie Soup
- Dinner: Celery Root Soup

Day 4:
- Breakfast: Mango and Spinach Smoothie
- Lunch: Baked Lemon Sole
- Dinner: Italian White Bean and Spinach Soup

Day 5:
- Breakfast: Pumpkin Spice Mousse
- Lunch: Grilled Mahi-Mahi with Pineapple Salsa
- Dinner: Fennel and White Fish Stew

Day 6:
- Breakfast: Almond and Apricot Bars
- Lunch: Grilled Octopus with Olive Oil and Lemon
- Dinner: Leek and Potato Soup

Day 7:
- Breakfast: Pineapple Carpaccio
- Lunch: Chicken and Mango Salad
- Dinner: Squash and Corn Chowder

Week 10

Day 1:
- Breakfast: Watermelon Pizza
- Lunch: Moroccan Chicken Stew
- Dinner: Sweet Potato and Coconut Soup

Day 2:
- Breakfast: Turmeric Latte
- Lunch: Spinach and Walnut Stuffed Chicken
- Dinner: Mushroom and Tarragon Soup

Day 3:
- Breakfast: Buckwheat Pancakes
- Lunch: Prawn Cocktail with Avocado
- Dinner: Zucchini Basil Soup

Day 4:
- Breakfast: Oatmeal with Berries
- Lunch: Herb-Crusted Halibut
- Dinner: Curried Cauliflower Soup

Day 5:
- Breakfast: Mixed Berry Salad
- Lunch: One-Pan Harissa Chicken
- Dinner: Celery Root Soup

Day 6:
- Breakfast: Sautéed Tempeh
- Lunch: Thai Coconut Shrimp Soup
- Dinner: Broccoli and Arugula Soup

Day 7:
- Breakfast: Mango and Spinach Smoothie
- Lunch: Baked Lemon Sole
- Dinner: Leek and Potato Soup

WEEKLY MEAL PLANNER + WORKBOOK

	BREAKFAST	LUNCH	DINNER	SNACKS
MONDAY				
TUESDAY				
WEDNESDAY				
THURSDAY				
FRIDAY				
SATURDAY				
SUNDAY				

Describe your current daily diet. What foods do you typically eat for breakfast, lunch, dinner, and snacks?

....

....

....

....

....

....

WEEKLY MEAL PLANNER + WORKBOOK

	BREAKFAST	LUNCH	DINNER	SNACKS
MONDAY				
TUESDAY				
WEDNESDAY				
THURSDAY				
FRIDAY				
SATURDAY				
SUNDAY				

What are your favorite foods and meals? Are any of these foods known to trigger your psoriatic arthritis symptoms?

WEEKLY MEAL PLANNER + WORKBOOK

	BREAKFAST	LUNCH	DINNER	SNACKS
MONDAY				
TUESDAY				
WEDNESDAY				
THURSDAY				
FRIDAY				
SATURDAY				
SUNDAY				

List any foods that you believe may exacerbate your psoriatic arthritis symptoms. How do you feel after consuming these foods?

....

....

....

....

....

WEEKLY MEAL PLANNER + WORKBOOK

	BREAKFAST	LUNCH	DINNER	SNACKS
MONDAY				
TUESDAY				
WEDNESDAY				
THURSDAY				
FRIDAY				
SATURDAY				
SUNDAY				

Have you tried any dietary changes in the past to manage your psoriatic arthritis? If so, what were they and how did they impact your symptoms?

....

....

....

....

....

WEEKLY MEAL PLANNER + WORKBOOK

	BREAKFAST	LUNCH	DINNER	SNACKS
MONDAY				
TUESDAY				
WEDNESDAY				
THURSDAY				
FRIDAY				
SATURDAY				
SUNDAY				

What are your primary goals for starting the psoriatic arthritis diet? (e.g., reducing inflammation, losing weight, increasing energy levels, etc.)

....

....

....

....

....

....

WEEKLY MEAL PLANNER + WORKBOOK

	BREAKFAST	LUNCH	DINNER	SNACKS
MONDAY				
TUESDAY				
WEDNESDAY				
THURSDAY				
FRIDAY				
SATURDAY				
SUNDAY				

How often do you currently consume processed foods, sugary snacks, or beverages? How might you reduce your intake of these items?

WEEKLY MEAL PLANNER + WORKBOOK

	BREAKFAST	LUNCH	DINNER	SNACKS
MONDAY				
TUESDAY				
WEDNESDAY				
THURSDAY				
FRIDAY				
SATURDAY				
SUNDAY				

Identify any potential barriers to following the psoriatic arthritis diet. How can you overcome these challenges?

WEEKLY MEAL PLANNER + WORKBOOK

	BREAKFAST	LUNCH	DINNER	SNACKS
MONDAY				
TUESDAY				
WEDNESDAY				
THURSDAY				
FRIDAY				
SATURDAY				
SUNDAY				

List three new recipes from the psoriatic arthritis diet that you are excited to try. What ingredients do you need to buy to prepare these dishes?

WEEKLY MEAL PLANNER + WORKBOOK

	BREAKFAST	LUNCH	DINNER	SNACKS
MONDAY				
TUESDAY				
WEDNESDAY				
THURSDAY				
FRIDAY				
SATURDAY				
SUNDAY				

Describe a typical grocery shopping trip. How can you adjust your shopping habits to better support your new diet?

....

....

....

....

....

WEEKLY MEAL PLANNER + WORKBOOK

	BREAKFAST	LUNCH	DINNER	SNACKS
MONDAY				
TUESDAY				
WEDNESDAY				
THURSDAY				
FRIDAY				
SATURDAY				
SUNDAY				

Identify any foods or ingredients that you are uncertain about regarding their impact on psoriatic arthritis. How can you research or test these foods?

....

....

....

....

....

....

WEEKLY MEAL PLANNER + WORKBOOK

	BREAKFAST	LUNCH	DINNER	SNACKS
MONDAY				
TUESDAY				
WEDNESDAY				
THURSDAY				
FRIDAY				
SATURDAY				
SUNDAY				

What are some dining-out strategies you can use to stay on track with the psoriatic arthritis diet when eating at restaurants or social events?

....

....

....

....

....

....

Scan the QR code below to get a surprise bonus!